THE INNER SOURCE

INNER THE SOURCE

EXPLORING HYPNOSIS WITH DR. HERBERT SPIEGEL

DONALD S. CONNERY

HOLT, RINEHART AND WINSTON
NEW YORK

Library of Congress Cataloging in Publication Data
Connery, Donald S.
The inner source.
1. Hypnotism—Therapeutic use.   2. Hypnotism—
Therapeutic use—Case studies.   3. Spiegel, Herbert X.,
1914-   .   I. Title.
RC495.C59   615.8'512   82-2882   AACR2
ISBN: 0-03-046496-X

First Edition

Printed in the United States of America
1 3 5 7 9 10 8 6 4 2

ISBN 0-03-046496-X

ACKNOWLEDGMENTS

The reader will find in these pages the names of those patients, physicians, and researchers whose contributions and encouragement have been essential to the making of this book. They have generously shared their knowledge and experience with us in order to advance the public's understanding of hypnosis. We thank them all.

Among the names is that of David Spiegel, but he provided more than information and inspiration. To the author, who came to see him as the best of that new breed of doctors who are alert to the self-healing powers of their patients, he has been a kind friend and wise counselor. To Herbert Spiegel, he has been not just a son but the closest of colleagues: "the person whose ideas and advice have had the greatest influence on my work."

CONTENTS

DIALOGUE *ix*

INTRODUCTION *xi*

1 Trance Talent *1*

2 Self-Control *12*

3 The Myths *28*

4 Aroused Imagination *41*

5 Discoveries *66*

6 Investigations *80*

7 The Columbia Course *98*

8 The Eye Roll *126*

9 The Profile *142*

10 Apollonians—Odysseans—Dionysians *158*

11 Personality and Hypnotizability *173*

12 No Smoking *184*

13 Mastering Symptoms *205*

14 Pain *233*

15 Future Trance *249*

DIALOGUE

PHIL DONAHUE: What's the point, Dr. Spiegel? Is it your view that hypnosis is a vehicle for healing?

HERBERT SPIEGEL: It can be a vehicle for healing if you structure it that way, but it's essentially a method of concentration that most of us have. It's a way of having a parallel awareness: being here and alongside yourself at the same time. This parallel awareness is an exquisite power that we have and therapeutically we can use it in many ways.

DONAHUE: Being a hypnotic subject or not being a hypnotic subject has nothing to do with intelligence, intuition, creative ability—or does it?

SPIEGEL: Yes, it does. People who have an impairment of their intelligence have great difficulty in concentrating this way. So it does require a certain degree of average or above-average intelligence. People who are highly hypnotizable are usually very imaginative. Their fantasy and imaginative life is so great that they can often make creative use of hypnosis. People who are low on the hypnotizability scale can be imaginative, but it isn't as poetic or as free-floating as the highly hypnotizable person.

DONAHUE: But all that notwithstanding, we're still not sure what hypnotism is, are we?

SPIEGEL: We're not sure of a lot of things. We don't know how aspirin works, but we still know how to use it. We don't know what electricity is, but there are an awful lot of things we can do with electricity.

DONAHUE: It's your view, then, that hypnosis ought to be used more than it is in therapy?

SPIEGEL: Yes. It's too bad that it's been ignored. In many ways we are indebted to the quacks and the vaudeville people who have been keeping this art form alive over the centuries because the scientists have been ignoring it for a long time. But since the 1930s and '40s there has been a gradual emergence of interest in hypnosis in science and medicine. We're now appreciating what the old-time doctors knew. And that is: As good as science is, as important as it is to use pills when appropriate, or surgery, we also have another powerful therapeutic agent, and that's our mind.

INTRODUCTION

During the writing of this book, the popular CBS program "60 Minutes" reported on the surging interest in hypnosis in the United States. "Its use for minimizing suffering may just be starting," said correspondent Dan Rather. "The leading expert in the country, perhaps in the world, is Dr. Herbert Spiegel, Clinical Professor of Psychiatry at Columbia University's College of Physicians and Surgeons."

As these words were spoken, Dr. Spiegel, a genial-looking man with a trim black mustache and a Kojak-like shaven head, was seen on film with a young woman who happened to have an exceptional gift for the trance state. Spiegel was about to demonstrate hypnotic age regression for medical professionals at a special course on hypnosis given at the University of Miami, one of the many institutions where he has lectured on the uses of trance in treatment.

The physicians, surgeons, dentists, psychiatrists, and psychologists gathered there had already learned from Spiegel that people with the ability and the desire to focus their minds and take the plunge into the trance experience may well be able to employ hypnosis for a variety of therapeutic ends. It is useful for pain relief, for anxiety and insomnia, for smoking and weight problems, for dealing with any number of habits, phobias, and psychogenic illnesses, for easier childbirth, for removing fear before an operation and speeding recovery, for enhancing memory and improving skills, for mastering many difficulties of everyday life, and for the sheer pleasure of relaxation and meditation.

According to Spiegel, most people—nearly three quarters of the population—are hypnotizable to a clinically significant degree. They are perfectly able to make use of hypnosis as a creative instrument. Not only are they endowed with trance capacity to some measurable extent, but their good mental health permits them, in his words, "to maintain the ribbon of concentration" that is essential to hypnosis. Of the 30 percent or so who cannot be hypnotized, some simply lack trance talent, but many more are unable to utilize the trance talent they have. Psychological disorders keep them from maintaining concentration.

About 15 percent of the population are blessed, and sometimes cursed, by extraordinary trance talent. As the high scorers on Spiegel's zero-to-five scale of hypnotizability, they are known as "Fours" and "Fives." These hypnotic virtuosos account for much of the anecdotal material in the literature on hypnosis. The young woman sitting with Dr. Spiegel in the Miami auditorium, as seen in the "60 Minutes" film, happened to be one of them.

She was capable of such total movement into another state of consciousness that she could be regressed to earlier times in her life, relive them vividly, and then have no memory of the experience afterward—as Spiegel was about to demonstrate. "This technique," Dan Rather explained, "is said to be useful in psychotherapy to bring out forgotten childhood traumas that might be causing emotional problems later."

Spiegel had already asked the woman to put herself into a trance. In seconds, she became exquisitely attentive and receptive. She had wiped out all distractions and was focused exclusively on the doctor's instructions.

Telling his patient that she was no longer her present age but was getting younger and younger, Spiegel guided her to early childhood. "You're three years old," he said. "One year old. Six months old. *Today you are one month old.* Is there anything special today?" She gave no answer. There was no response to anything he said. But when he touched her cheek with his finger she moved her mouth toward it and began to suckle.

It was as if all memory of her life, except for the first four weeks, had been blocked off. And yet, because hypnosis is very greatly a matter of "being here and alongside yourself at the same time," as Spiegel so often says, the woman's internal monitor—the "hidden observer" that hypnosis researchers speak of—was standing by, keeping watch. Her parallel awareness enabled her to behave as the infant she once was while simultaneously remaining alert to the doctor's directions to move forward or backward in time.

When Spiegel suggested that she advance to her sixth birthday, she immediately began speaking of a little girl's concerns in a little girl's voice. She described the happenings of the day and complained: "I don't like where I live. There's nothing to do and everybody's fighting all the time."

Later, when signaled to return to the present, she emerged relaxed and refreshed from her hypnotic time machine.

What did the millions of "60 Minutes" viewers make of all this? Because hypnosis or hypnotism has been wrapped in so much mystery over the centuries and shadowed by so many myths and misconceptions, it is a good guess that many people seeing Herbert Spiegel in action concluded that he is a master hypnotist: a modern wizard with power to control the human mind.

Dr. Spiegel would be the first to disagree. Neither he

nor anyone else who is said to be expert in hypnosis projects any kind of exclusive power. Unlike Mandrake, the
Shadow, and other fictional characters, hypnotists possess
no magical means to "cloud men's minds" and impose a
superior will. Strictly speaking, a hypnotist does not hypnotize, and so it follows that Spiegel—a doctor who has
guided tens of thousands of patients and other persons
into the hypnotic state in the course of four decades as a
clinician and teacher—does not think of himself or call
himself a hypnotist.

In his view, all hypnosis is self-hypnosis. All that any
"hypnotist" does is tap the natural capacity of an individual for focusing, for concentrating, for imagining, for
visualizing, for blocking out distractions, for increasing
awareness, for achieving greater control over the body's
involuntary functions, for entering a different order of
consciousness.

The individual, in short, is not given anything new; he
is simply helped to engage the means he already possesses
in order to alter attention and perception and to influence his emotional and biological reactions. The trance
state he enters and enjoys is not so new or so extraordinary an experience as it appears to be. Most of us spontaneously go into trance far more often than we realize.
Unknowingly, we use this special state of mind to good
advantage. It is beneficial to be able to concentrate so
totally on a task or a good book or a favorite piece of
music that we are oblivious to normal distractions. Someone who is daydreaming or lost in thought seems to be in
another world—so much so that we often ask, "Where
have you been?"—but we do not associate this with hypnosis because we see no hypnotist.

Even in formal hypnosis, when the so-called hypnotist
leads his subject into the trance state, no piercing gaze,
glittering watch, authoritative voice, or optical illusion is

necessary. The subtle shifting of mental gears requires no elaborate ceremony. Unless he has been trained in old-fashioned techniques, a doctor who goes through a dramatic ritual in order to induce hypnosis may do so only because he thinks it is more effective with patients who expect something like the antics of stage hypnotists.

By turning on his trance capacity, with or without the guidance of a hypnotist, the individual clears the channels for the kind of interior communication that may lead to a solution or a cure or a way to make better use of his or her resources. Hypnosis puts us in touch with ourselves. It is a pathway to the inner mind. It is a means for igniting our built-in powers for self-healing. If most of us have not consciously made use of our trance ability, it can only be because we remain unaware of the possibility. "Hypnotic capacity is part of our makeup," Spiegel points out, "and hypnosis goes on a lot of the time anyway, so why not use it to reach a personal goal?"

It was Spiegel who discovered the link between vertical eye mobility and hypnotic potential. The extent to which we roll our eyes upward tells more about our natural bent for the trance state—and about our personality as well—than we imagine. This finding, made in the early 1960s, has been substantiated by thousands of cases.

An apparently fixed biological indicator, the eye roll serves as a telltale sign of hypnotic ability for everyone who is sound enough in mind to maintain concentration. The trance-limited "Lows," as Spiegel calls them, show little eye movement when asked to look all the way up while holding the head level. In sharp contrast, the trance-talented "Highs" display such eye mobility that we see a lot of sclera, or white tissue, as most of the iris disappears beneath the upper eyelid. The eye-roll measurement is made when the patient, upon the clinician's request, slowly closes his eyelids while continuing to gaze upward. What counts is the distance between the lower eyelid and the lower edge of the iris. (For a chart showing the range of eye roll, see Chapter 8.)

For the medical professional, the eye roll is just the starting point in a more detailed assessment—Spiegel's Hypnotic Induction Profile—of a patient's potential for using hypnosis in therapy. The Profile is something new in the world of medicine: the first practical clinical means for determining hypnotizability. It is a five-to-ten-minute test that invokes a trance under monitored conditions, permits observation of motor responses, and draws from the subject a report of his or her sensations. And, because the Profile reveals whether a patient is mentally "intact," it can serve as a diagnostic probe as well as a guide to the most suitable psychotherapy.

In Spiegel language, the people on the high side of the scale of hypnotizability (the Fours and Fives) are the more emotional, imaginative, and trusting *Dionysians*. Chameleonlike in their reactions as they quickly pick up cues and easily identify with the joys and sorrows of others, they seem made for hypnosis. In fact, they spend much of their time in trance without realizing it. They tend to dwell in the present, giving little thought to the past or to plans for the future. Their excellent memories can be a boon—especially for the student who may be able to recall whole pages of a textbook at examination time—but their readiness to suspend critical judgment can lead to trouble.

Those on the low side of the scale (the Zeros and Ones) are the more rational, quizzical, and skeptical *Apollonians* with little or no trance ability. Valuing reason over passion, thinking a lot about the past and future as well as the present, they cherish control and are reluctant to accept new ideas without scrutiny. They are more likely to be found among attorneys and accountants than among actors and artists.

The majority of people, including Spiegel and the author, are *Odysseans* (the Twos and Threes) with mid-range eye rolls and Profiles. They are a blend of the extremes. Sometimes the Odysseans seem as head-oriented as the Apollonians, while at other times they display the heart-oriented qualities of the Dionysians.

For all of these character types, motivation must be married to trance talent if hypnosis is to be used creatively. An Apollonian with enough ambition to quit smoking or lose weight, for example, may more successfully use his limited trance capacity for leverage than a less-motivated Dionysian who has trance talent to spare.

In the closing years of his life, Reinhold Niebuhr, the renowned theologian, suffered several strokes that left him with a persistent pain in his lower intestinal tract as well as a painful and spastic left wrist and arm. He found it agonizing to sit down and work at his typewriter, yet he was determined to carry on his activities. Because analgesics and physical therapy gave him only partial relief, he gladly took up a medical friend's suggestion that he talk to Dr. Spiegel about possibly overriding the pain with self-hypnosis. When Spiegel called on him, he said that he understood what was involved because there were times he became so "hypnotized" by a thought or a subject that he could temporarily "forget" the pain. Although low in trance capacity, he succeeded in forgetting the pain for longer stretches of time and was able to get more work done with less agony.

"His desire to continue working," Spiegel says, "made him a good hypnotic subject. He was also a good student with a genuine interest in hypnosis. I had to go to his bedside and, frankly, I was in awe of the man. He was a great thinker; a great philosopher. Who was I to tell him what to do? Fortunately, I thought of something Will Rogers had said: that we're all ignorant, only in different fields. He got a kick out of that. I told him, 'This is one area where I think I know more than you do, so I'm going to ask you to be the pupil and I'll be the teacher.' He was delighted to learn something new.''

This kind of meeting of minds characterizes Dr. Spiegel's work in hypnosis. He is a teacher more than he is a hypnotist. He does not hypnotize patients so much as he introduces them to their innate ability to hypnotize themselves. He teaches them to understand, appreciate, and utilize their trance capacity. Viewing trance as an art form, he offers hypnosis as a creative exercise—and he is frank to say that he has learned more about hypnosis from his patients than from any other source.

Once a patient has discovered his gift for hypnosis, Spiegel bows out early. He does not encourage the belief that he must be consulted repeatedly. Sometimes a follow-up is called for, but he usually sees patients only for a single session. Once they have found their trance ability and learned a treatment strategy to deal with their problems, they are on their own, fully capable of summoning their powers of mind. Success with hypnosis, he suggests, will be their success, not his.

Spiegel remembers with delight the Florida woman whose husband sent her to him in order to cure her phobia about dogs. The man said the last straw came when he was entertaining important business clients in an elegant restaurant, and his wife sent the food and wine flying. She had leaped up in terror at the sight of a white poodle. The woman proved to be a mid-range hypnotic personality, and used her trance talent to restructure her perspective toward dogs. In a few weeks she overcame her fears so totally that she talked to her husband about getting a dog of her own. She was upset, however, when he thanked Spiegel for her new lease on life. "I'm the one who deserves the credit!" she protested. "She was absolutely right," Spiegel says. "She did it herself once she learned that she could use self-hypnosis for self-mastery."

Inasmuch as this book is about Dr. Spiegel but not by him, I need not be reticent in describing his position in international hypnosis: It is unique. He is a psychoanalyst who turned from analysis to more direct forms of psychotherapy long before most of his contemporaries. His career has coincided exactly with the flowering of medical hypnosis in the last forty years. "The dogma of psychoanalysis," Spiegel says, "is that you can't evoke changes in people unless you understand why. Much can be done with hypnosis without knowing why."

As the discoverer of the eye roll and the developer of the Hypnotic Induction Profile (HIP), he is an innovator who has made it possible, at long last, for medical professionals—who are inclined to think of hypnosis as "too unscientific"—to make it part of their everyday practice. As a clinician who measures what he does and as a hypnosis investigator who conducts his research in the real world of patients, he is exceptional in bridging the twin disciplines of clinical and experimental hypnosis.

Now in his sixties and uncommonly vigorous (he jumps fences on his appaloosa hunter three days a week, several hours each time), Spiegel has been tapping the trance capacities of his patients ever since 1942, when he was the first American psychiatrist to go into combat in World War II and the first to return home wounded. A Columbia University clinical professor for many years, and more recently a special lecturer, Spiegel's annual postgraduate courses on basic and advanced medical hypnosis at Columbia Presbyterian Medical Center in New York have trained a small army of clinicians in the recognition of trance talent and in its therapeutic uses. While carrying on a busy private practice in Manhattan, he finds time every year to appear at hospitals, medical schools, and scientific conferences as a kind of Johnny Appleseed of clinical hypnosis, forever encouraging physicians to look to the mind as well as the body.

I first met Herbert Spiegel because of a murder. In September 1973, in a small town close to my own home in Connecticut's Litchfield Hills, an eighteen-year-old named Peter Reilly arrived home one night to find his mother's battered and mutilated body on the bedroom floor, the last of her blood draining from a gaping throat wound. He frantically telephoned for help. The State Police arrived within minutes and took him into custody. In the course of an exhausting eight-hour interrogation by four officers, which stands as a prime example of psychological coercion, the confused youth agreed that he must have been the one who killed his mother. "It really looks like I did it," he said, even though he had no memory of the event. His signed confession led to his arrest, five months in jail before trial, a jury's guilty verdict, and a long prison sentence.

Dr. Spiegel played a vital role in overturning this classic and nationally publicized instance of injustice. He came into the case at the behest of playwright Arthur Miller, the most prominent of the Connecticut citizens who were seeking a new trial. At the same time, I was beginning my research for a book on Peter Reilly's fate, *Guilty Until Proven Innocent*.

In a confrontation with the prosecutor that was worthy of a Perry Mason thriller, Spiegel appeared as a surprise witness at the hearing for a new trial. Spectators, intrigued by his shaven dome, big bow tie, and orange-sherbet shirt, saw a man of average size and calm demeanor who spoke most respectfully, with professional precision, even when the prosecutor's questions were inane or insulting. The seriousness of the proceedings could not hide his rich sense of humor or his pleasure at having a hand in the demolition of the case against Peter. When asked by the prosecutor to name some medical schools other than Columbia where he had lectured, he tried not to smile as he mentioned Harvard, Yale, Stanford, Chicago, Cornell, Pennsylvania, NYU, Emory, Rome, "and several others I cannot recall."

By employing the Hypnotic Induction Profile as both a measure of hypnotizability and a diagnostic probe, Spiegel had determined that Peter Reilly had none of the characteristics of a person who spontaneously would shift into trance to such a degree that he would be unable to account for his actions afterward. Moreover, Spiegel had found that the youth's "serious deficit in his ability to identify who he is as a person," the result of emotional and psychological impoverishment, had made him singularly vulnerable to the pressures of police interrogators who asserted—falsely—that they had "proof positive" of his guilt and demanded that he confess to the crime. Spiegel was able to destroy the police and prosecution claim that amnesia accounted for the teenager's inability to provide the details of a murder that he had not, in fact, committed. His explanation of the reasons for Peter's false confession was so lucid that Judge John A. Speziale, who is now Chief Justice of the Connecticut Supreme Court, told him: "You are the most credible expert witness that I have ever heard in my years on the bench and as a private attorney." The judge ruled that a "grave injustice" had been done and ordered a new trial. Within months, Peter Reilly was free of all charges.

I was in the courtroom during Spiegel's two days of testimony. Quite apart from having my interest in hypnosis stimulated, I sensed the value of the Profile test to the criminal-justice system. In addition to determining trance capacity and personality traits, it disclosed proneness to particular psychological disorders. Spiegel, in fact, has frequently been asked by prosecutors and defense attorneys, as well as the FBI and the Secret Service, to examine suspects and witnesses in criminal cases and to testify about his findings. He was recently appointed Adjunct Professor at John Jay College of Criminal Justice in New York.

Clearly, Dr. Spiegel was a man worth knowing. We became friends. We found that we shared a concern about police interrogation techniques and related criminal-justice matters. He had seen how careless questioning of witnesses to a crime, using hypnosis, can contaminate memories. He had shown how hypnosis, in the right hands, can be used to improve recall and provide leads to decisive evidence.

For my part, as a former foreign correspondent with experience in the Soviet Union and other police states, I had a built-in interest in the methods of mind conditioning that are popularly described as brainwashing. I was impressed that Dr. Spiegel did not offer the usual public relations response to the layman's inevitable question: Can a hypnotized person be led to say or do things contrary to his beliefs—even to lie, steal, or kill? While the answer is a reassuring no as a generality, Spiegel refuses to overlook the special vulnerability of exceptionally hypnotizable people to deceit and deception. A remarkable experiment of his own—filmed by NBC and described in Chapter 6—goes far to confirm that a programmed-to-kill "Manchurian Candidate" is at least plausible.

The more we discussed these matters, the more I realized that Spiegel's findings and opinions not only contradicted the popular mythology about hypnosis but challenged much of the established wisdom. It seemed to me that he was reinventing hypnosis. Other clinicians and researchers, many of whom had been his students, were moving in the same direction, but he was at the forefront of a movement to strip the subject of its old authoritarian trappings (the dominating, controlling hypnotist; the submissive, compliant subject) and offer it as a self-discovering, self-mastering experience suitable to a free and informed society. Above all, he was challenging the medical profession to pay more attention to a therapeutic modality, so often dismissed as outdated and unscientific, that may well be the most modern of all the tools of modern medicine.

As a means for engaging the protective and restorative mechanisms of the body, hypnosis appeared to be fundamental to the new—yet truly very old—approaches in medicine and psychotherapy that call on the troubled individual to bring into play his or her capacity for self-healing and self-improvement. While making my own initial inquiries into the nature of hypnosis, I came upon a recently published book, *Stress*, by Walter McQuade and Ann Aikman, which described the way Dr. Spiegel's patients maintain a cure for asthma attacks by using self-hypnosis. "It sounds not unlike meditation and biofeedback," said the authors, "and Spiegel himself agrees." He was quoted as saying, "Whether you attach electrodes to your head or listen to a priest in a saffron robe, it is all essentially the same. Call it Zen, acupuncture, TM, biofeedback, or Mesmer, it taps the same kind of attentive, narrowed inner concentration, erasing peripheral distractions—and it can be very useful."

I knew that Spiegel, in collaboration with his son and associate, Dr. David Spiegel, Assistant Professor of Psychiatry and Behavioral Sciences at Stanford University's

School of Medicine, had completed a landmark work on hypnosis for medical professionals, *Trance and Treatment.** Believing that a different kind of book for a wider audience was needed, I proposed that we do it together, combining my curiosity and his authority.

I wanted a free hand to write it in the manner of a reporter who had come fresh to hypnosis, as if to a new country, and had found in him an expert guide. I wished to attend his Columbia courses, sit in on sessions with patients, monitor his research, talk to his colleagues and other clinicians and experimenters, and question him at length about his life and work. My purpose was to clarify hypnosis by describing the adventures and discoveries of an explorer who had journeyed far into uncharted territories of the mind and who clearly believed, like the philosopher Don Juan in Carlos Castaneda's *Journey to Ixtlan*, that "We are as mysterious and as awesome as this unfathomable world, so who can tell what we're capable of?"

He was agreeable. And so we have this book. While it is intended to throw fresh light on a subject that has seen too much darkness, the reader should not take it as the last word. We are still learning the wonders of the human mind. As Spiegel tells the doctors he teaches, "The last word on hypnosis hasn't been written, and I don't suppose it ever will be. I have seen thousands of people in trance but I've never stopped being awed by what happens."

* New York: Basic Books, 1978.

THE INNER SOURCE

1

TRANCE TALENT

The fact that the mind rules the body is, in spite of its neglect by biology and medicine, the most fundamental fact we know about the process of life.
    —FRANZ ALEXANDER, *Psychosomatic Medicine*

We are our own best hypnotists.

Margaret Bourke-White, the great *Life* photographer, was once asked how a sensitive person like herself could bear to photograph the horrifying sights at Buchenwald at the close of World War II. "Sometimes I have to work with a veil over my mind," she explained. "When I photographed the murder camps the veil was so tightly drawn that I hardly knew what I had taken until I saw the prints of my own photographs."

Ernest Hemingway, describing the times when he was writing well, spoke of how "the wrist took over and the words just took wing." James Thurber, reflecting on the workings of his mind, said, "I never know when I'm not writing. Sometimes my wife comes up to me at a dinner party and says, 'Dammit, Thurber, stop writing!' She usually catches me in the middle of a paragraph. Or my daughter will look up from the dinner table and ask, 'Is he sick?' 'No,' my wife says, 'he's writing.'"

Jackie Stewart, the veteran champion of Grand Prix motor racing, has told of his sense of detachment when a race begins: "I see things through absolutely cold, crystal-clear eyes, without fear or apprehension of any kind. It's a strange feeling, a feeling of being totally removed from the scene and looking at it from the outside, as though I'm no longer a part of my body." And because so many complex calculations have to be made from moment to moment, "the greatest requirement is to eliminate the sensation of speed so that instead of a corner rushing up to you, it comes to you slowly and passively. For me, it's like watching a film in slow motion."

Arthur Miller, marveling at the way a great actor's imagination can be so strong that he becomes the character he is playing, has said that "he casts a shadow that is not his own." He remembers seeing Lee J. Cobb, after struggling to "get into" the role of Willy Loman in *Death of a Salesman*, "suddenly popping through that door and there he was and his name was Willy. Miraculous!" Miller says that he wept "with love of that art: the idea of being able to imagine oneself into a position like that."

When Carl Yastrzemski, the pride of Boston, came to bat in the last half of the ninth inning of the classic Yankees–Red Sox playoff game in 1978, he was aware only of "total silence," even though 34,000 fans in Fenway Park were screaming their heads off. At such a moment, he told a reporter, his mind is so focused that there are just two people in the ballpark: "Me and the pitcher. The crowd may be cheering or booing, but for me, it's as if they're not there. I analyze the situation—the pitcher's strengths, what he's likely to show me—and I concentrate."

None of the notables just described was hypnotized in any formal sense. No hypnotist put them into a trance. Yet hypnosis was happening just as surely as if each of them had knowingly used the trance state. Instinctively, these artists and athletes had reached into themselves for resources that lie in reserve. Their use of mind power may strike us as mind-boggling, yet what they did was by no means exceptional. Inasmuch as the great majority of us are endowed with trance capacity to some degree, the spontaneous combustion of concentration, imagination, and motivation has given us more frequent trance experiences than we realize. Our lives would be less rich and more difficult if we lacked the ability to become utterly absorbed in matters of compelling interest and to feel and imagine intensely. Recognition of our individual trance talent is the first step toward purposeful use of hypnosis.

Trance is a naturally occurring phenomenon. Hypnosis is simply its formal expression. Trance can take place whether one means it to or not. Slipping into trance is something that most people do from time to time all of their lives. "Our sense of awareness in everyday life," says Dr. Herbert Spiegel, "is a constant balance between focal attention and peripheral awareness. You go into trance when you increase your focal attention while reducing your peripheral awareness. You tune out distractions in order to concentrate.

"When a surgeon is absorbed in a delicate operation," Spiegel points out, "the odds are very great that he unwittingly goes into a trance state." We see trance at work when the infatuation of lovers makes them oblivious to everyone else. Trance ability permits the bored businessman at the opera to turn off the soprano so that he can play movies in his mind about his favorite fishing spot. In William Styron's *Sophie's Choice*, the heroine listens for a while to the droning of a preacher during a graveside service, and then "I began to tune him out as one cancels sound with the dial of a radio, allowing my mind to capture drowsily only the plumpest and moistest platitudes."

Trance is present when a character like Thurber's Walter Mitty weaves heroic fantasies while carrying on a conversation with his wife. Hallucination is a trance experience. A stage hypnotist can lead a subject to believe that there is a fly in his ear or water in an empty glass or one person sitting in two chairs at once. In like fashion, we can convince ourselves—especially if the circumstances are as hypnotic as the telling of ghost stories around a campfire—that we really do see a ghost or a flying saucer.

One of the most common manifestations of trance is called "highway hypnosis." You are driving at high speed on a busy turnpike. As you see the sign for your exit and begin slowing down in order to make the turn, you suddenly realize that you have no memory of the last half hour or the last thirty miles. Your mind was on other things, perhaps reviewing a speech or making plans for a holiday, yet you made all the curves and stayed a safe distance from other vehicles. The internal monitor who was doing the driving—looking after your safety while you dwelled on things far from the highway—is the same observer who stands by during hypnosis, silently keeping track of the proceedings. This marvelous parallel awareness, this divided consciousness, is the hallmark of the hypnotic experience.

The soldier who storms a machine-gun nest on his own, heroically oblivious to enemy mines and bullets, is probably in a trance state. Chroniclers of combat speak of battlefield euphoria, of a soldier's sense of the unreality of it all, of his feeling of detachment from danger, of floating above fear. Survivors of battles have told of their sensation of being spectators who watched themselves fighting, as if in a film. "The whole plan of attack flashed through my mind in a matter of seconds," writes Philip

Caputo of an incident in Vietnam in *A Rumor of War.*
"At the same time, my body was tensing itself to spring.
Quite separate from my thoughts or will, it was con-
centrating itself to make a rush for the tree line. . . .
Without a command from my conscious mind, I lunged
into the woods."

When a child's life is in danger or the house is on fire,
we suddenly find ourselves moving with extraordinary
energy, carrying great weights and otherwise displaying
strengths that we did not know we possessed. We are so
single-minded that nothing else matters, not even pain.
Once the emergency is over, we may feel the euphoria
that is common to hypnotic experiences. *Life* recently
told of a middle-aged woman who, with her husband,
won a Carnegie Hero Award for rescuing a man from the
flaming wreckage of his truck. Far from being exhausted
by the event, she said, "It's like having a baby. It's the
greatest feeling you can have. I can't remember feeling so
good about anything in my life."

Similarly, countless athletes, amateurs as well as professionals, have told of psychic ecstasy, mystical insights,
new levels of consciousness, or feelings of being swept
beyond the ordinary sense of self when they surpass
themselves at sport. Some speak of floating through a performance and of becoming so airborne that they watch
themselves, with awe, doing the seemingly impossible. "I
felt complete detachment," wrote Roger Bannister of the
race that broke the four-minute-mile barrier. Billie Jean
King has told of peak moments in tennis when "my concentration is so perfect it almost seems as though I'm able
to transport myself beyond the turmoil on the court to
some place of total peace and calm."

But is it correct to speak of such experiences, such
displays of trance phenomena, as hypnosis? Dr. Spiegel

makes a distinction between formal and informal hypnosis—or what might be called official and unofficial
hypnosis.

On the one hand, there is the formal, structured, inten-
tional ceremony for starting, using, and ending trance.
"The hypnotist knowingly induces trance," Spiegel says,
"maintains a sensitive contact with the subject during
the trance state, and then gives a clear cutoff signal to
come out of the trance state." Or else, in self-hypnosis,
the person who has learned to do so puts himself into
trance for some purpose and brings himself out of it in
response to his own signal.

On the other hand, there is the wide spectrum of
unwitting, spontaneous trance phenomena without any
starting and stopping ceremony. Spiegel customarily begins his basic hypnosis course for doctors by mentioning
a number of trance situations: everything from sleep-
walking, daydreaming, and fugue states to being in love
and becoming totally absorbed in a good book or film. He
sees hypnotic elements at work in the cures of faith healers and in the way a patient's suffering may be relieved by
a sugar pill, or placebo, that the doctor has described as a
painkiller.

Whether produced spontaneously or deliberately, the
trance state is an expression of a capacity for a different
order of consciousness that the individual may possess
without even knowing it. William James observed long
ago that "our normal waking consciousness, rational consciousness as we call it, is but one special type of consciousness, whilst all about it, parted from it by the
filmiest of screens, there lie potential forms of consciousness entirely different. We may go through life
without suspecting their existence; but apply the req-
uisite stimulus, and at a touch they are there in all
their completeness, definite types of mentality which

probably somewhere have their field of application and adaptation."

One of the best-known applications of trance ability is in pain relief. Most people, once they understand how to use the mind to direct the body, are able to reduce and perhaps even eliminate pain altogether. To Dr. Harold Wain, a psychologist who is a cofounder of the pain clinic at Walter Reed Army Medical Center in Washington, D.C., hypnosis "is a gift that the patient has. All I'm doing is helping him unwrap it, and helping him develop strategies that will allow him to deal more effectively with pain."

Like the ability to play the piano, Spiegel says, trance capacity is inherent. It is a natural endowment—and some people are more endowed than others. "To some extent it can be sharpened by instruction and practice, but one's capacity for hypnosis pretty much remains fixed in the adult years. A hypnotist merely helps an individual use a skill he already has. The individual, if he is hypnotizable, has the ability to sustain in response to a signal a state of attentive, receptive, intense focal concentration with diminished peripheral awareness. Hypnosis is a function of an alert person who utilizes his capacity for maximal involvement with one point in space and time and thereby minimizes his involvement with other points in space and time."

Such fine tuning of the mind can provide the occasion for flights of the imagination. Much has been written in recent years about the differing thinking and imagining styles of the analytical left brain and the intuitive right brain. Trance seems to put the left brain into neutral while the right brain does a solo performance. Arthur Koestler has said of the creative act that at the decisive stage of discovery, "the codes of disciplined reasoning are suspended—as they are in the dream, the reverie, the manic flight of thought, when the stream of ideation is free to drift, by its own emotional gravity, as it were, in an apparently 'lawless' fashion.''

According to Max Planck, the father of the quantum theory, the creative scientist must have "a vivid intuitive imagination for new ideas not generated by deduction, but by *artistically* creative imagination." Part of the artistry that produces a creative leap is the formal or informal trance process of focusing, floating, and letting things happen. It is a kind of mental free wheeling. Images and ideas appear "out of the blue." Many painters and composers have told of working in such an abstracted state of mind that they are amazed afterward to see what they have created. Many writers, from Shelley, Thackeray, and Wordsworth to Dickens, Goethe, and Stevenson (who gave credit to the "Brownies" who worked while he slept), have spoken of their best work coming from some place beyond consciousness.

"The trick in writing," says Robert Penn Warren, "is to get in a certain condition to have an idea. It won't come by logical manipulation. You have to learn the art of blankness." Saul Bellow, when asked by a reporter how he was coming with the Nobel Prize lecture that he was to deliver in Stockholm the following month, replied, "I like to do these things in a state of trance, but so far I haven't found the entrance."

Medical hypnosis is largely a matter of putting people in touch with their imagining powers for therapeutic purposes. While teaching hypnosis one day at Columbia Presbyterian Medical Center, Dr. Spiegel was told of an interesting patient who happened to be under treatment in the nearby dermatology clinic. He was a twenty-seven-year-old salesman with a twenty-one-year history of itching and scratching on his hands and legs, and of chronic skin inflammation. The salesman was invited to be seen by Spiegel in front of the assembled physicians. As a mid-range hypnotic subject, he responded well to instructions that he imagine a cool, tingling numbness in his hands and legs instead of the usual itching. He responded so well, in fact, that he said he not only could feel the tingling but "I hear bells ringing!" Later, during a discussion of his case, he exclaimed, "Do you doctors realize what has happened here? My itching is gone!" The salesman was taught how to use his trance talent to keep on controlling the symptoms. The itching and the inflammation were still gone when Spiegel contacted him four years later.

Another patient, a woman who frequently was embarrassed by incontinence, was asked to use her imagination during trance so that she would be able to project her troubles on a huge, personal movie screen and examine them at a distance. By floating *here* while putting her problems out *there*, she could free her body of the need to express her anxieties. The patient realized immediately that she could float and focus and imagine in this manner because she had recently done so on her own without thinking of it as self-hypnosis.

"I was riding in a crowded subway train on a hot summer's day," she told Spiegel, "and I began to get dizzy because of the heat. I had read somewhere that you could put yourself out of the immediate area if you concentrated hard enough, so I started picturing my Canadian childhood. I looked at myself walking to school when I was five years old. In my mind I went through the whole thing about putting on the boots and the mittens and the coat, going outside, walking in the snow, feeling the cold snow against my face and the way the cold hits you in the lungs when you take a breath. After five minutes of this my hands were cold. I looked around and everybody else was hot but I was very, very cold."

The importance of imagination in the hypnotic experience was illuminated a decade ago by a leading hypnosis researcher, Josephine Hilgard, the author of *Personality and Hypnosis: A Study of Imaginative Involvement*. Many intensive interviews with people who differed widely in their trance capacity led her to conclude that the hypnotizable person is "capable of a deep involvement and almost total immersion in an activity, in one or more imaginative feeling areas of experience—reading a novel, listening to music, having an ecstatic experience of nature, or engaging in absorbing adventures of mind and body." Dr. Spiegel, in developing the Hypnotic Induction Profile, had already found that the low scorers on his zero-to-five scale of hypnotizability were noticeably lacking in these personality features while the high scorers had them in abundance.

The total immersion of children in a game of "let's pretend"—when they carry on as if broomsticks are really swords and orange crates are really rocket ships—is akin to the deep involvement of a patient in medical hypnosis who vividly imagines, as the doctor has suggested, that there is a block of ice resting lightly on his head. The coldness makes his head feel so numb that he no longer feels the pain of his migraine headache.

The same trance power that permits fantasy and imaginative involvement can provide the means for greater achievement in work or play. The ability to concentrate is vital for anyone striving for excellence. When a performer goes into a slump or falls short of his potential, it is often said that he has "lost his concentration." Bobby Jones, the great golfer, once observed that he knew he was playing well when he thought of only one thing while making his shot—and he knew he was playing very well when he thought of nothing at all. Pelé has told of playing World Cup soccer games "in a kind of trance."

Accepting rather than questioning one's sensations is a key to the success of a trance experience. Explaining his ability to lose himself in the part he is playing, film actor Christopher Walken, a deranged soldier in *The Deer Hunter* and a ruthless mercenary in *The Dogs of War*, said, "There's a part of myself that operates very well if I just leave it alone. Most of us are better off not trying to figure anything out. You're never going to be as smart as that part of yourself that lets go."

It is no surprise that a leading investigator of mind-body phenomena, Marilyn Ferguson, finds that "Children are notoriously better than adults at biofeedback, almost certainly because they are too ignorant to know that they are attempting the impossible." To Zen master D. T. Suzuki, "Man is a thinking reed but his great works are done when he is not calculating and thinking. 'Childlikeness' has to be restored with long years of training in self-forgetfulness." For the trance talented, however, the long years are not necessary. The gift of hypnosis is there. It is not too farfetched to think of it as instant Zen: a switching on of one's auxiliary mental powers.

2

SELF-CONTROL

What is it then that hypnosis supplies that
does this extraordinary enabling, that allows
us to do things we cannot ordinarily do except with great difficulty?
                    —JULIAN JAYNES, *The Origin of
                       Consciousness in the Breakdown
                       of the Bicameral Mind*

Pamela, a beautiful actress, had been plagued by insomnia
ever since childhood. Recently, however, because of the
natural anxiety of any performer who goes from audition
to audition seeking a part in a play, her sleeplessness was
worse than ever. "I was in a state of desperation," she
remembers. "I was literally shaking from complete tired-
ness when I went to Dr. Spiegel's office. I went in there
desperately wanting help."

What happened in the next forty-five minutes changed
her life. Pamela learned that she had a definite and measurable talent for hypnosis—a talent she could use whenever she wished to separate herself from the worries that
were costing her so much sleep.

During part of her session with Dr. Spiegel she was
guided into the trance state. When she came out of it,
upon his signal, she had a wonderful sense of floating. She
felt relaxed and refreshed. She was delighted to know that
she could maintain or recapture this feeling of serenity

on her own through self-hypnosis. And yet she was also a little disappointed.

"Is that it?" she asked. "I expected something glorious. . . ."

Spiegel smiled. Some of his patients feared the worst about hypnosis, thinking that they would have no control of their own minds, while others had exaggerated expectations of instant salvation or a spectacular high. Some even complained, despite just having given a vivid demonstration of their hypnotic ability, that "nothing happened." They had not "gone under," they insisted, because they could remember everything that happened and every word that was said. They didn't realize that they were *supposed* to remember. That was the whole point of the exercise: to be deeply impressed by what they had felt and by what they had heard.

He said to Pamela: "You probably have a Hollywood idea about hypnosis. Here we do a Broadway version."

"I expected to be off into another world," she said, "but, in fact, I was not."

"Actually, you were off into your own world."

"Yes. And I loved it."

Touching her face, she realized that she had shed a few tears during the trance.

"That just means that you were really in touch with yourself," Spiegel said.

"I know. I felt very close to myself."

Hypnosis is a discovery experience. Pamela literally found herself. She discovered her capacity to deal with the forces that had kept her in such a state of tension. She learned how to let her body float. At long last, she could sleep.

"This feeling of floating," Spiegel tells his patients, "is something you can have around the clock. You've identified a natural phenomenon and learned the art of turning it on and using it yourself. If you leave here thinking that I did this to you, that would be wonderful for my ego but it would be a great big lie. You brought this capacity with you when you walked in the door, and it is quite within your power to keep on having this good feeling."

Like millions of other insomniacs, Pamela had tried everything she could think of to get a good night's sleep. Nothing worked. She had managed to put up with the problem most of her life, but when the tensions and frustrations of her career robbed her of all but a few hours of rest, she went to a psychiatrist to see if he could find a solution. After three months of exploration of her mental state and personal history, she still couldn't sleep. One day she asked the psychiatrist a question about hypnosis. He told her, "We'll have nothing to do with that!"

Nonetheless, Pamela obtained a book about hypnosis. "It wasn't a very good book," she says, "but I noticed that there were many references to Dr. Spiegel, so I decided to see him."

Spiegel's office is on the ground floor of an apartment building just off Madison Avenue on Manhattan's Upper East Side. It is a neighborhood of town houses, embassies, art galleries, restaurants, and several of the world's great museums. The office is a busy workplace. At any one time, Spiegel and his colleague, Dr. Stanley Fisher, may separately be seeing patients while in other offices researchers and secretaries carry on the compilation and analysis of data on hypnotizability and treatment results for long-range studies.

Once seated in a comfortable leather chair, Pamela gave Spiegel a brief account of her personal history and the nature of her insomnia. He was less interested in the "why" of her sleeplessness over the years than in her resources for gaining control over such a troubling symptom. Hypnosis began when he asked her to do an eye roll, which revealed that she was a Two-Three, and to relax and imagine herself floating. He took her through the several steps of his test for hypnotizability—the Hypnotic Induction Profile—before bringing her out of trance. Spiegel was now equipped with the knowledge that she was an intact or mentally healthy person with mid-range trance capacity. And he could see that her desperate desire to sleep normally would help her make the most of her hypnotic talent.

Again, Spiegel guided her into trance. In this alert and focused state of mind, she was ready for instructions, like an actress waiting for a director's orders. He says, however, that "I was more of a catalyst than a director. I showed her how to rearrange her resources so that she could do her own thing. It was simply a matter of showing her a way of distancing herself from her anxieties that had not occurred to her before."

He taught her the "screen technique." She was asked to visualize "a movie screen, a TV screen, or, if you wish, a clear blue sky that acts like a screen." She was encouraged to see it as a split screen so that she could put her problems on one side: "on your worry screen." Other thoughts and images could be placed on the other side. In short, this was her theater of the mind and she was both the projectionist and the sole member of the audience. If there were troubles in her life that were causing her tension and anxieties, those troubles could be put on the worry screen instead of being inflicted on her body. The worries would still be there, available for examination, but the body could relax. While she was still in trance, Spiegel told her that she would be able, by herself, to go into hypnosis at any time and use the screen.

Pamela headed home that evening feeling euphoric. She talked to her husband about the experience for three hours. Then, after a brief self-hypnosis exercise, she got into bed and fell asleep. She has since been able to sleep well. She still feels the pressures of her work; she still has anxious moments; but she can deal with them and put them in their place. The mere knowledge that she can master insomnia has brought a ripple effect that has changed other things in her life for the better.

Pamela was asked to be a guest at Spiegel's advanced course of hypnosis several months after her visit to his office. She agreed to come. He understood that hypnosis had helped her but had no idea of what her responses would be to the doctors' questions. When she appeared at the ground-floor auditorium of Columbia Presbyterian Hospital and realized that she was about to face a hundred psychiatrists, she had a jolt of stage fright. But, as she explained to the doctors a few minutes later, "the nice thing about self-hypnosis is that you can do it just like that! I sat down in the back of the auditorium and in two seconds I put myself into a little trance and became relaxed immediately. When Dr. Spiegel first told me about the eye roll I thought it was a dumb thing to do; I really did. I didn't know what it was about. But now I guess it has something to do with the actual state of trance because all I have to do is the eye roll and I'm off!"

With Spiegel serving as a straight man, letting her give her own account of things, Pamela entranced her audience. Lithe, vivacious, and strikingly dressed, she displayed an obvious intelligence that rebuked anyone who believed that only the weak-willed can be hypnotized. She said that she had responded immediately to Spiegel's view of hypnosis as a "personal art form." She explained that "I liked this a lot because that took it out of the cold, dry technique category. It becomes something that you can use in your own way. The good part about hypnosis is that you feel that you're doing it yourself and that's a nice feeling."

When asked about the worry screen, she said, "Oh, I use it all the time. Especially at night but during the day as well, I find that if I am able to place all of the concerns I've had up on the screen and allow them to do whatever they want to do, somehow it frees me from any responsibility for having to worry about those things. And the next thing I know I'm ready to go to sleep, and I have been sleeping very, very well without medication."

"Muscle tension is the enemy of sleep," Spiegel noted. "The typical insomniac keeps himself awake by fighting it, by telling himself to sleep. But ordering your muscles to relax is like speaking Chinese to your muscles. They don't understand it. Pamela learned that she didn't have to let her muscles reflect the anxiety. It wasn't a matter of denying that she had these worries, but she had a place for them out there on the screen. Instead of fighting the anxiety, she could say to herself something like this: 'I'm a person. I have many attributes. I have all sorts of things and I have worries too. I can put the worries over there instead of here. I'll deal with them later if I feel like it but right now I can float. My body can relax.'"

Said Pamela: "I use the screen a great deal. I use it almost always before an audition or something of that nature when I find I am nervous and uptight. It's not easy to deal with the realization that you are trying out for a part and you're probably going to be rejected. I feel that I'm able to get myself out of the problem and put it at a distance. I disassociate myself from it. And by doing that I feel as if I'm almost transcending what's happening. It's like I can really see what's going on and say, well, that's that and it really doesn't have a great deal to do with me. Or, if it does have a great deal to do with me, then *how* it does. It's helped me a lot."

"Pamela uses the labels just right," Spiegel added. "She distances herself. She doesn't deny the problem's there but by establishing the sense of distancing she's able to get a perspective on the problem. The overview enables her to enhance her sense of executive mastery over what she's doing."

One of the doctors asked Pamela to describe hypnosis. "It's just being able to focus in and concentrate on something," she said. "You just get your body in a state where you feel relaxed, then you do the eye roll, close your eyes, and that's it! At least it is for me. It's the way a road narrows as you look in the distance. You're focusing on that one thing and enjoying the view. I don't think about anything; I just do it. Sometimes at home I make it more of a ceremony and make it last longer. Before my husband comes home, to be more relaxed with him, I'll have a little trance ceremony. It has helped our relationship in a lot of ways."

This, of course, was one manifestation of the ripple effect. She spoke of being "more aware of my dreams; more conscious of what I dream about." Then she mentioned something that she thought truly astonishing. "For many years I tried to wear contact lenses but I could not adjust to either soft or hard lenses. I just couldn't adjust, period. Since my session with Dr. Spiegel, I've gone back to the doctor and I've been wearing soft contact lenses ever since. I can't explain it except to say that one day the concept of contact lenses came up out of nowhere. All of a sudden, on the right side of the screen, I saw something to do with my eyes and with contact lenses. I zoomed in on it and I said, aha, I can wear these things and I'm going to. And I did!"

As a final thought, Pamela told the doctors: "It isn't as if I no longer have any difficulties. I still have anxieties. Since seeing Dr. Spiegel I have had two or three nights of restless sleep but compared to what I was going through before, it's like night and day. The main thing for me is that I no longer feel like a victim."

"You give up control to gain control," Spiegel says. "The great paradox about hypnosis is that what appears to be a loss of control is really an exercise in greater control."

In medical hypnosis, the patient, by relaxing and letting go, by shifting into an accepting and unquestioning state of mind, becomes extraordinarily receptive to the doctor's suggestions and directions—and, later, to his own instructions in self-hypnosis. They are received loud and clear, without static and with the kind of clarity that we associate with "moments of truth," and they make a deep impression on the mind. In turn, the mind wields a profound influence over the body, even to the point of affecting normally involuntary processes. There is often a reduction in blood loss when hypnosis is used in place of chemical anesthesia during surgery.

Hemophiliacs, or "bleeders," have been able to take hypnotic control of nosebleeds and avoid excessive blood loss during dental surgery. Dr. W. L. LaBaw of the University of Colorado Medical Center has done pioneering work with hemophilic children, using "suggestive therapy" in group sessions to show how to relax and rely on trance to reduce pain and bleeding. One of LaBaw's case histories, as reported in the medical journal *Haematologia* in 1970, concerned a teenager whose blood disorder had sent him to the hospital many times a year for most of his life, often for prolonged care. On one occasion, just the act of biting his tongue necessitated seventeen days of hospitalization. The boy's schoolwork suffered because of his distress over his infirmity, LaBaw said, and he sorely needed to regain a sense of personal worth.

"He learned to mobilize his idle trance capability," La-Baw explained, "becoming an ardent disciple of that method of relaxing. His academic performance began to mirror his intellect, greatly improving as he lowered his level of stress by using his suggestibility. Many weeks passed without his need for the hospital. A coagulation time near normal was eventually obtained, the lowest in his record." When the youth went for eight and a half months before returning to a hospital for treatment (feeling pain in his right knee at a time of great tension over an impending college entrance examination), it represented "by far his longest remission in nineteen years of struggle" and "roughly an 800 percent improvement over the five just previous ones. During a week in the hospital, other forms of treatment than transfusion, including suggestive therapy, were successful. Up to the time of this report, he has not required another inpatient stint, having been in the hospital one time in the past thirteen months. Though bleeding tendencies are known to improve spontaneously, this patient's use of his suggestibility is thought to deserve part of the credit for his startling remission. He accomplished it by minimizing the effect of the 'psychophysiological mechanism superimposed upon the physical defect' which is recognized in bleeders."

Despite the vast literature on the uses of hypnosis to influence physiological processes that once were considered involuntary, and to cure or control such afflictions as warts, rashes, asthma, and allergies, many doctors could not bring themselves to accept the information until the outpouring of data about biofeedback during the last two decades.

Because a biofeedback machine reports with tones,

lights, or graphs the degree of self-regulation, it was clear that an individual can, like an Indian yogi in deep meditation, slow down his pulse and heartbeat, reduce muscle tension, raise and lower skin temperature, increase and decrease blood pressure, control brain-wave frequency, and more. Biofeedback, like hypnosis, has been used for everything from the relief of migraine headaches to the control of premature ventricular contractions by heart patients. In the words of one laboratory volunteer: "It's as if your body has always been on automatic pilot and suddenly you find you can take over the controls."

Taking over the controls, but without the need for a machine, is what hypnosis is all about. Once a patient discovers his idle trance capability, as Dr. LaBaw expressed it, and links it to a treatment approach for his particular problem, he takes charge of his own healing. As has happened countless times in Dr. Spiegel's experience, the cigarette smoker frees himself from the habit by deeply absorbing a fresh outlook, as proposed by the doctor during the trance state, about his responsibility for protecting his body from poisonous smoke. The pain patient, giving flight to his imagination as the doctor suggests, finds that he is able to turn off the agony. The stutterer, relaxed and floating as he is encouraged to speak rhythmically instead of rushing his words, talks normally for the first time in years.

Although the patient can be said to be under the doctor's control while in the trance state, it is control by permission and it is all to the purpose of guiding the patient toward the exercise of greater self-control. The hypnotized person does what the hypnotist suggests but all the while a part of him monitors the proceedings, makes sure that nothing untoward takes place, and delights in his own achievements.

"If I go to a French restaurant with someone who is an

authority on food and wine," says Spiegel when asked about the influence of the hypnotist, "and I leave all the ordering to him, with the result that I only eat and drink what he recommends, have I really surrendered control to him? I can always get up and walk out—just as the person in hypnosis can break off the trance if something offends him—but I like what is happening. For the objective of a good meal I let him take over. I enjoy a wonderful dinner. I'll know what to order the next time when I'm on my own. So who is controlling whom?"

The parents of a pretty twelve-year-old girl brought her to Spiegel's office one day to see if hypnosis could somehow put an end to her thumb-sucking habit. Despite numerous efforts to deal with the problem, she had been sucking her thumb so constantly for so long that her teeth were coming loose. Major dental work was in prospect. The patient was seen by Spiegel's associate, Dr. Barbara DeBetz, who measured her trance capacity and found that she was on the high side of the hypnotizability scale. The girl's own statements indicated considerable trance talent: "I do a lot of daydreaming. I get lost in things." Fortunately, she was also strongly motivated to get rid of her habit. She was tired of being teased about it by her schoolmates.

As expected, she went swiftly and deeply into trance. The essence of Dr. DeBetz's message to her was: "You are your body's keeper and you alone have full control over what you put into your body." She was told that thumb-sucking is an insult to her body. She needed her body to live. She owed her body respect and protection. Self-hypnosis could be her way of protecting her body by controlling any impulse to suck her thumb.

DeBetz showed her how to put herself into a quick little trance every few hours in order to remind herself of her new viewpoint about her body and her ability to take charge of herself. As DeBetz learned afterward, the patient mastered her thumb-sucking immediately and soon was able to forgo the reinforcement of her regular self-hypnosis exercise. The habit was still absent when an inquiry was made a year later.

In another case, a young Javanese woman and her American husband traveled halfway around the world to see if Spiegel could help her conquer her fear of flying. They were a newly married couple. As an oil executive based in Singapore, he had looked forward to his wife's company on his frequent business flights around the Orient. He was dismayed to discover that she would panic at the very thought of going up in an airplane. A Chinese doctor recommended that he take her to Spiegel. The executive arranged to have her placed under sedation and carried aboard an aircraft on a litter. He flew with her to New York.

The Hypnotic Induction Profile test revealed that the woman was a Three-Four: a better-than-average candidate for hypnosis. After leading her into trance, Spiegel proposed that she adopt a whole new perspective about her relationship to the airplane during a flight. He explained that she could use her gift for trance to overcome her anxieties and replace her usual feeling of helplessness with a sense of mastery—as if she herself were at the controls of the aircraft. He taught her a self-hypnosis strategy that she could use in future flights to "float with the plane" instead of fearing the plane. The floating feeling that hypnosis can produce is a kind of transcendence: a sense of repose and well being, a rising above ordinary concerns.

At the close of the appointment, the husband mentioned that his wife also had a phobia about bridges and tunnels. He was worried about what would happen if they went ahead with plans to visit relatives in New

Jersey. Spiegel said that the trance strategy she had learned to deal with her fear of flying could be applied in other situations. Her trance ability was part of her nature; it was something she could turn to at any time to put herself at a distance from her tensions and fears.

As Spiegel was informed soon afterward, the couple hired a car and drove to New Jersey and back to Manhattan—by way of the George Washington Bridge and the Lincoln Tunnel—without any difficulty. A letter from Singapore some time later told him that his patient was so relaxed during the long flight home that she slept most of the way.

As these cases demonstrate, hypnosis in therapy, after the initial session with the clinician, is most often a matter of the patient using the trance state on his own—acting as his own therapist—to make sure that he responds to the directions he gives himself. "The value of hypnosis," Spiegel will tell a patient, "is that it makes your mind optimally receptive to your own thoughts."

A young concert pianist, for example, sought help because his anxieties during a performance, especially his fear of forgetting the score, were distracting him so much that he was unable to play at his best. Spiegel introduced him to his trance capacity (as a Two he was about average), showed him how to hypnotize himself ("You can give your mind the same kind of clarity that you sometimes get by floating in a bathtub"), and taught him a technique for separating himself from his worries. "The answer to your performance anxiety," Spiegel said, "is not to say, 'Don't be nervous.' That's as dumb as saying, 'Don't think about having an itch on your nose' or 'Don't think about swallowing.' You are bound to be nervous about performing. You can deal with it, however, by shifting into trance, imagining a huge movie screen, and putting your anxieties out there on the screen while you remain here, on the stage, concentrating on your performance."

Another patient presented Spiegel with the opposite problem. He was an actor who had always counted on the "butterflies" in his stomach to get him keyed up for a performance. Then one night, apparently because he had become bored with the play, he had no anticipatory anxiety. "I turned in the worst performance of my life," he told Spiegel. "Now I want to know how I can get my butterflies back." He was taught a trance strategy that he could use before a performance to give himself the keen edge and anxious alertness that he felt he needed.

Because performing artists as a group are more hypnotizable than others, many of them manage to master personal and professional problems with their trance ability without realizing that hypnosis is at work. One actor who appeared at Spiegel's Columbia course—to describe how he had used trance to conquer insomnia—said that when he first started acting, and had been on a stage for only the fourth or fifth time, "I felt something shifting, and that whatever I was doing was coming from my subconscious mind rather than being anything I had planned before." He said that this natural trance "gives you a sense of complete isolation. You're solitary. At the same time, you hear noises. You know what's going on around you. You're not really out of touch with reality but the fact that there are people out there doesn't matter. The cues are all coming from the inside."

Commented Spiegel: "This is a beautiful description of a reduction of peripheral awareness to facilitate focal attention. All we're doing as clinicians is describing these natural experiences in more systematized terms and helping people understand what is going on. If they know that they are using their trance capacity, then perhaps they can do it better, just by having this extra knowledge about it. If you have a sailboat with an auxiliary engine, it's great to be able to put that engine on when you need it, when the sails aren't helpful enough. If we think of trance as an auxiliary engine, many people have it but don't know it. Sometimes it goes on and off without their intending it to go on and off. It can get pretty mischievous if you're trying to manipulate your sails in the wind and the engine suddenly starts. What you need to know is that it's there, how to identify it, how to control it consciously, and how to make the best use of it."

One conscious use of trance can be seen in a hospital labor room when a mother-to-be relies on hypnosis instead of chemical anesthesia to take care of any discomfort. Extraordinarily receptive to suggestion, she accepts the doctor's proposal that she see herself relaxed and happy and feeling good as she floats in the warm water of a Caribbean resort. She locks this image in her mind so that she can keep on floating and enjoying herself while the delivery of her baby proceeds. If there is pain, she is indifferent to it because it has no place in her beach scene, and yet she is not so removed from reality that she is unaware that she is giving birth. Indeed, she is alert and aware of events to an extent unknown to the woman who has been drugged to free her from pain.

As the doctor describes what is happening and as she sees the child immediately upon delivery, she is, in some miraculous way, in two places at once: in a hospital room and at the seaside. By creative use of her trance talent, she has achieved such a degree of control over her body that she has made the exhausting experience of giving birth an occasion of joy.

Other women have accomplished the same thing, in much the same way, without knowing that they were in trance. The natural childbirth teachings of Grantly Dick Reed, the Lamaze Method, and other breathing, relaxing, and imagining techniques have far more to do with trance—with hypnosis—than their advocates are prepared to admit.

The same can be said of meditation, acupuncture, biofeedback, est, faith healing, visualization methods, the Relaxation Response, Silva Mind Control, Suggestology, and other self-healing and self-awareness techniques. Many of the books published in recent years on new ways to enhance mind power read like carbon copies of old works on hypnosis, though they avoid any mention of trance or hypnosis. Thus, one book on visualizing the "movies in your mind" instructs readers to concentrate on breathing and "focus your attention on an imaginary spot in the center of your forehead. When your eyelids become strained and uncomfortable, let them drop. Notice the feeling of relaxation flow down."

In their book *Beyond Biofeedback*, Drs. Elmer and Alyce Green of the Menninger Foundation note: "Almost all of the popular commercial mind-training programs use a heavy dose of hypnotic programming. It may not be called hypnosis, and in fact it may be vehemently denied by instructors, but nevertheless many of the courses use hypnotic techniques that are 'right out of the book.' "

3

THE MYTHS

I mesmerize you all with this foolishness: my poetry and predictions and TV shows and sixteen-room mansions. Then you'll be listening when I say what I mean.

—MUHAMMED ALI, statement to the press

What accounts for the reluctance to call hypnosis hypnosis?

"Myths," said Salustius in the fourth century, "are things that never happened but always are." Myths about hypnosis are rampant. Doctors like Herbert Spiegel have had to contend with them throughout their years of effort to establish hypnosis as a commonplace medical tool. The toughest myth to put down is the belief that people who possess the secrets of hypnotic power can take over our minds and bend us to their will.

In Morley Safer's "60 Minutes" office in New York there is a framed letter from a viewer mounted on a wall. Insisting that "this is to be checked out without fail," the writer discloses that a certain woman still living in California sank the *Titanic*, kidnapped the Lindbergh baby, started World War II, helped the Japanese bomb Pearl Harbor, and assassinated President Kennedy, all through "the mighty power of mass hypnosis."

Though few of us are likely to think of hypnosis as

that powerful, we have been brought up to regard a hypnotist as a mind controller and to believe that to be hypnotized is to be helpless. In Eugene O'Neill's *Mourning Becomes Electra*, Orin tells his mother that her lover "was the one who planned father's murder. You couldn't have done that! He got you under his influence to revenge himself! He hypnotized you!"

For most people, the name that leaps first to mind when hypnosis is mentioned is Svengali. When the Los Angeles Police Department, seeking to get as many details as possible from witnesses to crimes, arranged for a number of officers to be trained in hypnosis, the headline writers promptly dubbed them "the Svengali Squad." While it is true that Svengali used his supposed hypnotic powers to enslave an innocent artist's model, it is also true that he never existed. He was only a creature of an author's imagination: the villain of George Du Maurier's novel *Trilby*, published in 1894.

Since then, an endless succession of cheap novels, comic strips, radio serials, and film and television dramas have conditioned us to be wary of hypnotism. One recent paperback, *The Hypnotist*, warns readers of the "awesome power" of the main character, a mad physician: "First he will relax you. Then he will heal you. Then he will try to bend you to his dark, malevolent will."

The idea of hypnosis as a mischievous and even menacing force became rooted in the public mind largely because almost everyone knew it only in terms of the bizarre behavior that a stage hypnotist or an experimenting college student could evoke from a hypnotized person. The stage hypnotist was adept at choosing as his subjects those members of the audience who were the most compliant, the most hypnotizable. After moving them into the trance state with a few strange words and gestures, he could get them to swat at a nonexistent insect, feel no pain when stuck with a pin, leap about the stage like monkeys, remain stiff as a board while suspended between two chairs, and so on. Witnesses to these activities were likely to believe that a hypnotist could make a person in trance do anything. All sorts of abuses could be imagined.

The sensationalizing of hypnosis was not offset by a public awareness of its value as a vehicle for healing and self-improvement. For a time, in the 1800s, hypnosis, while highly controversial, seemed to be on its way to acceptance by organized medicine. By this century, however, it was in eclipse. The comeback of medical hypnosis did not begin until the 1930s when an innovative young psychiatrist named Milton Erickson "almost single-handedly," in Spiegel's words, "reintroduced the use of hypnosis in modern medicine." It was slow going, however, until the outbreak of World War II. Then, military psychiatrists found hypnosis to be a most effective means for treating soldiers with war neuroses. Time was too short and the numbers were too great for the luxury of psychoanalysis and other forms of long-term therapy. Hypnosis provided a shortcut to the repressed memories that, in many cases, had to be acknowledged and examined before a mentally wounded GI could recover.

In the early postwar years, a number of dentists became interested in hypnosis for pain relief; so, too, did obstetricians who encouraged natural childbirth. Though comprising only a small percentage of practitioners, doctors in other medical specialties turned to hypnosis in their treatment of psychosomatic illnesses. In time, physicians and scholars engaged in clinical or experimental hypnosis founded the professional societies that flourish today. In 1958, three years after a similar move by its British counterpart, the American Medical Association endorsed the teaching of hypnosis in medical schools and its cautious use in medical practice.

The swelling interest in hypnosis inspired *Life* in 1960 to describe the "spectacular renaissance" of a medical tool that had long been "consigned to the cabinet of curiosities along with the leech and ipecac bottle." Aldous Huxley predicted that "within a few years, every city and village in North America may have its medical or dental hypnotist."

Life exaggerated and Huxley was premature. It is true, however, that two decades later there is greater interest in and employment of medical hypnosis than ever before in history. When the *Reader's Digest* published an article in January 1980 about the way clinicians like Herbert Spiegel use trance in treatment, the American Society of Clinical Hypnosis, one of the three professional societies listed as sources for the names of reputable hypnotherapists, was deluged with twelve thousand requests for information.

Although some turn to hypnosis more often than others, more than ten thousand physicians, dentists, psychologists, and psychiatrists in the United States employ hypnosis as a clinical tool. Thousands of other doctors, while not identified with hypnosis, use relaxation techniques and other hypnoticlike methods to ease the anxieties of their patients, give added thrust to treatment, and accelerate recovery.

The courses and workshops for clinicians conducted by the major hypnosis professional societies are more popular than ever, and there has been a steady rise in the number of medical and dental schools teaching hypnosis. More and more hospital administrators are recognizing the value of doctors and nurses being proficient in activating the trance capacity of their patients. The *Boston*

Globe, after learning that medical hypnosis is well established at such leading institutions as Massachusetts General Hospital, Beth Israel Hospital, and Harvard University Health Services, commented that "conservative Boston has hugged hypnosis to its stethoscope."

In a recent article, *The New York Times*, describing the movement of hypnosis into the mainstream of therapy in America, told of its increased use for everything from nail biting to the treatment of emotionally based symptoms that are common to victims of multiple sclerosis. (One clinician found that even some real neurological problems of the disease, such as loss of bladder control, can be relieved with hypnosis.) Therapists at the University of California at Los Angeles were turning to hypnosis to relieve the pain of terminal cancer patients, thus allowing them to remain alert and free of drugs. At Minneapolis Children's Hospital, researchers using hypnosis to treat bed-wetting were obtaining a cure or significant improvement in 80 percent of cases.

Although some clinicians who have made hypnosis a central part of their practice describe themselves as hypnotherapists, many more people with limited medical training, if any, also offer their services as hypnotherapists. Hypnotherapy is a term Spiegel considers unfortunate. Trance is not treatment, he says, and hypnosis by itself is not therapy. When a person comes to a clinician seeking help, it takes little skill to bring on the trance state but considerable skill to make a correct diagnosis, decide whether hypnosis is the best therapeutic means to employ, and then carry out beneficial treatment.

There is an obvious difference between a health-care professional who turns to hypnosis when appropriate and a hypnotist who knows only hypnosis. Some of the hypnotists who advertise in the newspapers and the yellow pages limit themselves to smoking, weight control, relaxation, and study and work habits. Others venture into areas best left to those who are trained in physiological and psychological processes. Because, in most states, anyone can practice hypnosis without being required to show proof of competency as a health practitioner, those seeking help should proceed with caution. Geographic listings of competent, ethically-bound clinicians can be obtained from the medical and psychological societies—the American Medical Association, the American Dental Association, the American Psychiatric Association, the American Psychological Association—as well as the primary hypnosis organizations.*

"It is not surprising that hypnosis attracts quacks," Spiegel says. "Medical history is largely the story of quackery flourishing wherever organized medicine failed to satisfy a need."

Inasmuch as a greater understanding and use of hypnosis, by doctors and patients alike, is impeded by mythology, Spiegel finds it necessary, when teaching medical professionals, to talk about ten of the most common beliefs. He does so in this fashion:

1. *Myth: Hypnosis is sleep.* In fact, hypnosis is the opposite of sleep. The individual in trance is not only fully awake but exceptionally alert, attentive, and responsive. After the trance, he usually remembers everything that took place. The calm, sleeplike look of the trance state is deceptive; in reality, the mind is focused and ready for what comes next. Electroencephalogram (EEG) studies

* These latter groups are: the American Society of Clinical Hypnosis, 2400 East Devon Avenue, Des Plaines, Illinois 60016; the Society for Clinical and Experimental Hypnosis, 129-A Kings Park Drive, Liverpool, New York 13088; the International Society of Hypnosis, 111 North Forty-ninth Street, Philadelphia, Pennsylvania 19139.

disclose that none of the brain-wave findings of sleep is present during hypnosis. The trance state provides a high incidence of alpha activity, revealing that the brain is resting yet alert.

We can hardly be blamed, however, if we have thought of hypnosis as a form of sleep. Hypnotized people give the appearance of sleep. Their eyes are usually closed because this facilitates concentration. They are peaceful, relaxed, and undisturbed by ordinary distractions. And, historically, authorities on the subject have related hypnosis to sleep.

The sleep myth has long been reinforced by the traditional terminology of hypnotists who chant, "You are going to sleep. A deep sleep. You are going deeper and deeper." Later on, their subjects are told to "wake up." While many modern hypnotists no longer talk about sleeping and waking up, they may still believe that with enough effort the trance can be "deepened." Spiegel is satisfied that an individual, unless he is resisting hypnosis or senses the uneasiness of the hypnotist, goes rapidly to his own trance level and no further. He dismisses the idea of deepening as "another hangover from mesmerism that is sheer nonsense."

2. *Myth: Hypnosis is projected onto the individual.* In fact, the hypnotist projects no kind of force or magic. All he does is tap the natural capacity that people have to experience trance. He does not have to pretend to possess special powers. Nor must he play the part of a commanding authority figure who can bend people to his will by sheer force of personality. No one who is hypnotizable and who is ready for hypnosis needs to be overwhelmed by the hypnotist. It is sufficient for the hypnotist to open the door, so to speak, so that the subject can step through on his own.

Despite the modern doctor's awareness that it is the

patient's trance capacity that is being engaged and not any mental force of his own that is being projected, he may well take credit for the trance or blame himself if there is none. In Spiegel's words: "Believing that eliciting a trance state involves projecting some quality of authority or control, a clinician will often be frightened when he meets an extremely compliant subject who seems almost ceaselessly plastic in responsiveness. Eventually this clinician is bound to run across a number of nonhypnotizable subjects and he would then assume that he had failed in some way. Either extreme implies taking more responsibility for what occurs in the trance condition than the operator has a right to do, and it confuses the diagnostic assessment."

3. *Myth: Only mentally weak or sick people are hypnotizable.* In fact, the opposite is true. The capacity to be hypnotized is a statement of relative mental health. In general, Spiegel says, highly intelligent and better-educated persons are more hypnotizable. While it is true that some perfectly normal people cannot be hypnotized, it is also true that schizophrenics, psychopaths, and others with serious mental or neurological problems cannot achieve the kind of sustained concentration that is essential to hypnosis.

Every physician experienced in the field is familiar with patients who believe that only the weak-willed can be hypnotized. Even if they have initiated the appointment with the doctor in order to give hypnosis a try, their first words are likely to be, "No one can hypnotize me!" Such defiance suggests that the patient is already concentrating so much on the business of being hypnotized that it may not take much to bring on the trance state. As in judo, the hypnotist can take advantage of that defiant force.

4. *Myth: Hypnosis occurs only when the hypnotist de-*

cides to use it. In fact, spontaneous or unintended trance experiences are far more common than hypnosis elicited by an expert. Spiegel's view is that the trance state is on a continuum with our normal waking consciousness. People with trance capacity slip in and out of trance more often than they know.

Highly hypnotizable persons, especially under stress or duress, are likely to shift into the kind of extreme trance states that come to a physician's attention. Most doctors recognize hysterical symptoms but too few realize that these are, very often, spontaneous trance states of highly hypnotizable individuals. In fact, most doctors are unaware of the extent to which they have a hypnotic influence themselves as authority figures dealing with patients who are yearning for a cure or an answer to their problems. Writing in the *Journal of the American Medical Association (JAMA)*, Dr. H. Clagett Harding, a Portland, Oregon, internist, said: "In my opinion, every physician is using hypnosis every day to varying degrees, and every patient goes into spontaneous hypnosis several times during the course of treatment."

5. *Myth: Symptom removal means a new symptom*. In fact, this is not necessarily so. Any number of troubling symptoms, from skin rash to fear of animals, can be successfully treated with the help of hypnosis without the appearance of a substitute symptom. Many symptoms are actually psychological fossils: remnants of earlier emotional times that linger on as habits. "Of course," says Spiegel, "if a doctor believes that another symptom is bound to appear, and if he conveys this conviction to a compliant patient, the patient will do what the doctor says. He'll produce a new symptom."

The symptom-substitution myth springs from orthodox psychoanalytical principles. Analysts closely wedded to Freud's belief that any neurotic symptom has its roots in unconscious conflict have been wary of removing a psychologically determined symptom too early in treatment. So long as the basic conflict remains, they have thought, another symptom will erupt in place of the one removed.

In Spiegel's experience, this just doesn't happen. To the contrary, patients who are able to master a symptom through hypnosis come out of the experience with a greater sense of well-being instead of a substitute symptom. Every so often, one of Spiegel's fellow psychoanalysts will call him into a case to help a patient get rid of a symptom before continuing with the long-term effort to get at the emotional roots—and then inform him later that the patient's freedom from his affliction brought about such a change for the better that the analysis was soon and successfully completed.

6. *Myth: Hypnosis is dangerous.* In fact, there is nothing dangerous about hypnosis by itself. If there were, we would certainly know it. We would have to tell ourselves not to slip into another state of consciousness, not to daydream, not to concentrate deeply, not to become totally absorbed in things of compelling interest. From a background of thousands of cases, neither Herbert nor David Spiegel can think of a single instance of adverse effects caused by the trance state. To the contrary, they are accustomed to patients reporting their enjoyment of the buoyant repose of this special state of mind.

Like anything else, of course, hypnosis can be misused by the careless practitioner or the unscrupulous layman. The heightened suggestibility and trusting character of the hypnotized person can be exploited, but it hardly needs saying that scoundrels can take advantage of people without hypnosis. In Spiegel's view, "it is the use to which hypnosis is put that counts, not the state itself. Hypnosis is a neutral state of attentive concentration. If a therapist introduces a therapeutically wrong proposal or unethically exploits the patient, then, of course, harm may result."

The most important "danger" of hypnosis lies not in its commission but in its omission. Physicians, on the whole, fail to take account of the trance capacities of their patients, and fail to consider using a medical tool of proven value that in many circumstances is unrivaled in its effectiveness. Patients who have become dependent on prescription drugs may be able, through hypnosis, to get along without them altogether. As a natural means for healing, hypnosis is not addictive, produces no injurious side effects, and is always available to anyone with trance talent.

7. *Myth: Hypnosis is therapy.* In fact, healing is accomplished *in* hypnosis but not *by* hypnosis. As already stated, hypnosis by itself is not therapy. Just as anesthesia can provide a setting for surgery, hypnosis serves as a matrix for treatment.

"Hypnosis alone is not a profession," Spiegel says. "Hypnosis is always secondary to a primary professional commitment. A dentist or a surgeon may use it to alleviate pain just as a psychotherapist may use it to implement appropriate behavior change, but these are not people who call themselves hypnotists. They are professionals who use hypnosis. There's no big deal about being a hypnotist. Anyone using that as a title is really making a statement about how limited his abilities are. He knows trance but what does he know about therapy?"

8. *Myth: The hypnotist must be charismatic, unique, or weird.* In fact, a flamboyant or eccentric personality might well disturb the trusting atmosphere that serves to bring out a person's trance talent. A patient who thinks his doctor is a zany character or a showman is less likely to ease into the desired state of relaxed concentration.

The old belief that a hypnotist is the possessor or pro- jector of some kind of secret force has obscured the truth that no special personality or special talent is necessary to hypnotize people. Virtually anyone can be a hypno- tist. The techniques of formal hypnosis are simple and quickly learned. Not so quickly learned are the therapeu- tic uses of the trance state. Spiegel's courses for medical practitioners are mainly concerned with the assessment of hypnotizability and with treatment strategies. Little time is spent on the business of eliciting trance. He tells the doctors, in mock dismay: "It is pretty frustrating for me to realize after nearly forty years doing this that to- morrow you will be able to go out and tap a person's capacity for hypnosis as well as I can."

9. *Myth: Women are more hypnotizable than men.* In fact, the sexes are the same in their trance capacity. Spiegel's work over four decades confirms the findings of numerous studies that disprove the notion of greater fe- male "susceptibility" to hypnosis. In his view, "The abil- ity to experience hypnosis is an example of real equality of opportunity for men and women."

Measurements of the trance ability of thousands of people seen by Spiegel and his associates, using the Hypnotic Induction Profile, challenge the old assump- tions about men being more rational and tough-minded and women being more emotional and impressionable. Women have long been characterized as prone to hys- teria. Some of the early investigators of hypnotic phe- nomena associated hypnosis with the state of mind of the hysterical female. Spiegel, however, has found that there is little difference in the percentages of men and women who are extremely hypnotizable and thus more likely than others to display hysterical symptoms. In much the same proportions, men and women run the gamut from the analytical and less compliant Apollonians to the intuitive Dionysians who are so responsive to a hypnotist's suggestions.

10. *Myth: Hypnosis is only a superficial psychological phenomenon.* In fact, hypnosis is at least as much a neurophysiological as a psychological phenomenon. For many years, experts in the field carried on a long and heated debate about whether hypnosis was strictly psychological. We now know that hypnotic capacity is associated with certain patterns of brain functioning, such as alpha waves on the electroencephalogram. After a searching review of hypnosis research, Kenneth Bowers, a leading scholar in the field, stated in *Hypnosis for the Seriously Curious* that "it is becoming increasingly clear that hypnotic susceptibility and its correlates are deeply imbedded in a person's biological organization. This is undoubtedly one reason for the relative stability of hypnotic susceptibility in mature people."

Spiegel's discovery of the eye roll, linking trance ability to the upward movement of the eyes, has provided fresh evidence that hypnosis is, in his words, a neurological phenomenon with a psychological overlay. An individual's trance capacity, he is convinced, either is present at birth or becomes a fixed part of the personality very soon afterward. It is still not clear whether this ability is inherited, is imprinted soon after birth, or is a combination of genes and early experience. Though there is some loss of hypnotic capacity as the years roll by—which permits the general observation that children are more hypnotizable than adults—a person who scores as a Low on the hypnotizability scale remains a Low all his years and a High remains a High.

No amount of practice or training will significantly enhance one's hypnotic ability, if any, Spiegel says. "Like an ear for music or any other natural gift, you have what you have, and that's it."

4

AROUSED IMAGINATION

> In spite of the remarkable power of hypnosis
> to reveal the inner mind and to direct both
> mind and body by the commands of a will
> obedient to thought alone, the unparalleled
> potential of hypnosis melted into the archives
> of psychiatry as scientific attention turned
> elsewhere.
>
> —BARBARA B. BROWN, *Supermind*

In *Shadows on the Grass*, a collection of stories about her
days in Africa, Isak Dinesen tells of a young Kikuyu
woodsman whose leg was crushed by a falling tree. His
fellow workers dragged him out from beneath the tree
and laid him on the grass. Dinesen sent a runner to get a
car so that the youth could be driven to the hospital.

"Kitau was lying in a pool of blood," she writes. "His
leg had been smashed above the knee and was sticking
out from his body at a grotesque and cruel angle." Weeping because of the great pain, he begged Dinesen for
"some of the medicine that helps people." All she had to
give to him were bits of sugar that she kept in her pockets
for the plantation animals. The sugar seemed to relieve
his agony but her supply soon ran out.

Once again he begged her for anything to stop the pain.
She remembered that she had with her a letter from the
king of Denmark thanking her for a lion skin that she
had sent him as a gift. She told the youth that she had
something "very excellent indeed. I have got a letter from

a king. And that is a thing which all people know, that a letter from a king in his own hand will do away with all pain, however bad." She placed the king's letter on his chest and her hand upon it.

"It was a very strange thing," Dinesen writes, "that almost at once the words and the gesture seemed to send an effect through him. His terribly distorted face smoothed out, he closed his eyes. After a while he again looked up at me. His eyes were so much like those of a small child that cannot yet speak that I was almost surprised when he spoke to me."

The youth was no longer in agony. He told her that the king's letter was indeed excellent and to please keep holding it on his chest. After the car arrived, she continued to hold it in place all the way to the hospital and into the operating room.

Word quickly spread about the power of the king's letter. "Soon they took to carrying up those of their sick who were in bad pain, so that they might have the letter laid on them and for a while be relieved. . . . No ache or pang could hold out against it."

Call it what you will: magic, faith, belief, imagination, suggestion, superstition, the placebo effect, mumbo jumbo. To Dr. Spiegel, what happened to Kitau was hypnosis. He has seen its like time and again in his office, in hospitals, on the battlefield, and in everyday life. The young African's reaction to the king's letter resembles the way many of us respond when handed a prescription by the doctor. As Norman Cousins observes in *Anatomy of an Illness*, "Most people seem to feel their complaints are not taken seriously unless they are in possession of a little slip of paper with indecipherable but magic markings. . . . The doctor knows that it is the prescription slip itself, even more than what is written on it, that is often the vital ingredient for enabling a patient to get rid of whatever is ailing him. Drugs are not always necessary. Belief in recovery always is. And so the doctor may prescribe a placebo in cases where reassurance for the patient is far more useful than a famous-name pill three times a day." No wonder, then, that for many years a high point of Spiegel's hypnosis course for doctors has been a lecture by Dr. Arthur K. Shapiro, the world's foremost authority on placebos.

Throughout human history, the most powerful medicine of all has been the faith of the patient in the healer and in the effectiveness of the treatment. In ways we are only beginning to understand, that unseen medicine of the mind sets in motion the self-healing mechanisms and chemical processes of the body. A doctor's bedside manner—warm or cold, sympathetic or indifferent—can profoundly influence a patient's attitude and encourage or discourage the healing activity. Indeed, it has been said of certain great physicians that they can make people feel better just by appearing at the bedside. Hippocrates observed that "some patients, though conscious that their condition is perilous, recover their health simply through their contentment with the goodness of the physician."

Environment can also influence a patient's ability to use his resources for healing. Norman Cousins attributes much of his recovery from a crippling disease to his move, with his doctor's consent, from a hospital where he was treated like an object to a hotel room where he felt a greater dignity and spent his time reading humorous books and watching comic films.

An article by Frank J. Mac Hovec in the *Journal of the American Society of Clinical Hypnosis*, describing ancient examples of hypnoticlike techniques, spoke of the Babylonians and their concern for a positive healing milieu: "They took their sick to the marketplace where they remained throughout the day, reclining on pallets. Friends, neighbors, and passers-by would stop and confer with the patient. If they had similar ailments they would offer advice and suggestions to encourage and reassure the patient. The repetitive nature of these suggestions planted the idea of recovery in the patient's mind, bolstering his hope, and reinforcing it in much the same way modern-day hypnotists approach behavior modification."

Attitude and atmosphere, so fundamental to healing, are basic to hypnosis. Long before he came upon the eye roll or put together the Hypnotic Induction Profile, Dr. Spiegel determined that the hypnotic trance comes about in a three-stage process, beginning with the *aura*, a distinctive atmosphere and frame of mind.

He describes the aura as a "series of expectancies and anxieties that the subject brings to the hypnotic situation. It can serve to enrich or maximize the hypnotic experience, as in a situation where the subject has been led to believe that this hypnotic encounter will result in the successful resolution of a major life problem. Or it can hamper the hypnotic experience as in a situation where the subject suspects that the operator will employ this trusting posture to exploit him."

The subject's desire for change or a cure and his anticipation that hypnosis will help him leads to the next stage: the *enhancement*. Here the hypnotist directs the patient's attention to the workings of the body. He might, for example, use a traditional trance-induction method and ask him to stare at an object held above the line of sight. He will suggest that the patient's eyelids are getting heavier and heavier—so heavy that his eyes must close. It is only natural, however, for fatigue to set in when one looks upward long enough. If the hypnotist asks him to fix his gaze on a dot on an otherwise blank sheet of paper, the predictable result is diplopia: The single dot becomes two dots, then one again, then two, etc. Similarly, it is only natural to feel light-headed or heavy-lidded while gazing at a light or a whirling disk.

"When the hypnotist tells the subject that his eyes are getting so heavy that he will have to close them," Spiegel says, "he is simply using natural physiological sequences and allowing the person to identify with them and accept the plausible interpretation that these events are occurring because of the message from the operator."

Impressed by the hypnotist and fascinated by what is happening, the subject moves on to the third stage: the *plunge*. Having already reduced much of his normal scanning awareness, he now shifts into such a state of concentration that he employs his maximal trance capacity. He is in hypnosis. The plunge may take the form of focusing on a sense of floating or a feeling of lightness in one arm or a heaviness in the legs, depending on what has been suggested. Now that peripheral distractions have been removed, the subject is supremely receptive to suggestion.

Spiegel describes this final stage of hypnosis in terms of the relationship between a swimmer and his coach: "The coach can guide the swimmer to the edge of the pool, can give instructions about how to jump, can even anticipate the actions in the water, but at some point the swimmer himself has to take the plunge into the water. The nature of the tie that the swimmer has with the coach can determine the ease, the speed, and the confidence that the swimmer has in exploring the water."

The three steps into trance—aura, enhancement, plunge—can most clearly be seen when the traditional trance-induction methods of hypnosis are used. They are many and varied and often quite time-consuming. Hypnotists used to put great stock in the monotonous repetition of sleep suggestions, or in a prolonged look-deep-into-my-eyes exercise, or in complicated movements of the hands that were called "passes." These rituals were believed to be necessary for eliciting hypnosis until it was discovered that a subject could be led into trance without seeing the hypnotist or even being in the same room with him.

In one legendary experiment, a hypnotist made a recording of his usual trance-induction monologue to see if his voice alone would do the trick. He asked his subject to take a seat, turned on the phonograph, and quickly left the room. Sure enough, when the hypnotist returned some time later the person was in a trance. He then discovered that he had, by mistake, put on a recording of Swiss yodeling.

On a number of occasions, Spiegel has hypnotized patients on the telephone—which is to say that even at long distance he was able to help them turn on their trance talent. In the case of the lady from Singapore, her husband telephoned him a year and a half after she had learned how to master her flying phobia to report that they had a problem. While his wife was doing a self-hypnosis exercise to prepare for her latest airplane trip, he said, he had accidentally knocked over a vase that was one of her favorite possessions. The noise had startled her out of the trance, she had become upset about the broken vase, and she had since found it impossible to go into trance and recapture the floating sensation that allowed her to feel comfortable when flying. "He wanted to know whether it was necessary for her to go all the way back to New York to see me," Spiegel relates. "I told him, 'Let's try it on the phone.' He got on another line while I talked to his wife so that he could tell me what was happening. I repeated the induction procedure with her and after a minute or two I could hear her saying, 'I got it! I got it!'

Then her husband said that she was in trance all right and that it looked like she would have no trouble going on the trip with him."

The patient who has trance capacity and wishes to be hypnotized, says Spiegel, does not have to be tricked into the trance state—as some of the traditional induction methods will do—or subjected to a lengthy ceremony. He needs only to be encouraged to relax, focus, and float, thereby putting his trance capacity to work. Spiegel's Hypnotic Induction Profile is an extraordinarily brief test for hypnotizability largely because the induction phase is quick and simple—as quick as it takes the subject to look all the way up, to close the eyelids slowly while continuing to look up, to take a deep breath, to exhale, to let the eyes relax while keeping the lids closed, to let the body float, to begin to feel sensations of floating.

Those who do self-hypnosis with these same steps can go into trance in a matter of seconds. The person with modest trance capacity who continues to check out his surroundings even as he enters hypnosis may not be so completely committed to the trance experience as someone with a greater natural ability, but each will reach his particular trance level with impressive speed. In fact, it may happen so quickly that the three stages of hypnosis just described will be compressed, as they are in spontaneous trance experiences.

On occasion, the hyped-up expectations that constitute the aura will be so great that the patient not only zooms instantly into trance but evokes the desired therapeutic response. Spiegel recalls a patient he was asked to see during a Sunday lecture on hypnosis at Emory University Medical School in Atlanta. The young woman was confined to a wheelchair because of hysterical paraplegia. All other approaches had failed and she was anxious to try hypnosis. As a fundamentalist Baptist, however, she was unsure whether it was proper to seek such treatment on the Sabbath. Fortunately, her minister assured her that a healing on Sunday would be "to the greater glory of God." The patient was so "psyched up," to use a valuable popular expression, that when she was wheeled into the auditorium and brought within twenty feet of Spiegel, she rose from the wheelchair and walked toward him. Her paralysis was gone (and gone for good, as he learned later on) before he could say a word.

And so it has been throughout human history. Infused with faith, their bodies aroused by great expectations, people have often brought about their own cures without knowing it. Credit would go to the medicine man or to the gods or to objects that were believed to be magical. People of the Stone Age carried scraps of bone, teeth, and the vertebrae of snakes in amulet bags because they were reputed to have the power to cure. Isak Dinesen's Africans were so enthusiastic about the king's letter as a cure-all that it was soon reduced to shreds. The pieces were secured in a leather pouch that a sufferer could wear about his neck. There are those in our own society who swear by the curative powers of copper bracelets or pyramid-shaped pendants.

Because imagining a cure can often accomplish a cure, much of medical history is the story of practitioners who employed various means of psychological persuasion to focus the minds of their patients and ignite their imaginations. Hypnosis was never discovered or invented; it was just given a label. Shifts of consciousness, trance experiences, and rituals of suggestion and compliance have existed for as long as human societies have existed.

The chants and ceremonies of shamans, witch doctors, and medicine men served as trance inductions and psychotherapy. The meditation rituals of the Chinese were designed to keep the so-called vital life force flowing freely from nature into the body and back to nature in a continuous circle. In ancient Babylonia, Egypt, and Greece, those who were sick in mind or body could find solace and perhaps a cure in "sleep temples."

Hypnosis has been a vital ingredient of every religion that has stressed healing through touch and prayer. The "laying on of hands" could work wonders with those whose ailments and afflictions were psychologically based—and who came to a healer in such an entranced state of mind that a word or a touch or the very atmosphere would suffice. For more than seven hundred years, the anointed kings of France and England had a celebrated "royal touch" that was believed to be better than any medicine. There were also charismatic figures who attracted great followings. They were the precursors of present-day faith healers and cult leaders who are said to have a hypnotic influence over their devotees.

Then, late in the eighteenth century, there appeared a superstar of healers: Franz Anton Mesmer, an Austrian physician (and friend of Mozart) who became famous for his magnetic cures. Wrongheaded as he may have been about the reasons for the success of his ministrations, Mesmer did an important service in demonstrating the value of trance in therapeutic work. Histories of hypnosis usually begin with Mesmer because he tried to provide a scientific explanation for trance phenomena (his ideas were based on Newton's law of gravitation) and because his activities touched off a great and lasting interest in the subject. He was such an original that his name became a label. He gave birth to mesmerism, which later became known as hypnotism.

As the author of a bold thesis on *The Influence of the*

Stars and Planets on the Human Body, Mesmer pro-claimed that there is a universal magnetic fluid flowing through everyone and everything. The startling cures he achieved were the result of his ability to harness this "an-imal magnetism," or so he believed. He attracted much attention when he restored the sight of the director of the Munich Academy of Sciences. Soon after this success, he was asked to look at an eighteen-year-old girl, well-known for her musical skills, who had gone blind fourteen years earlier when she was alarmed by a noise at her bedroom door. Mesmer had no trouble curing her of her hysterical blindness, as it would be called today. But when her parents arrived at his clinic to take her home, she refused to leave him. The mother slapped the girl. When Mesmer intervened, the father drew his sword. The mother fainted and the girl went blind again. Her sight was restored for the second time but only after she was left alone with Mesmer in the clinic.

The scandal of it all, the rumors of magnetic seduction, and the rising hostility of Vienna's medical establishment, forced him to move to Paris. He found the city to be delightfully open-minded and eager to give animal magnetism a try. Mesmer's hypothesis about an unseen universal fluid seemed to be perfectly in accord with the other invisible discoveries of the age: Newton's gravity, Lavoisier's caloric, Franklin's electricity, and the heated gases that were sending daring Frenchmen into the air in balloons. Louis XVI and Marie Antoinette were impressed by mesmerism. Others who were discontented with the academic and political establishment were glad to show their enthusiasm for a radical and irrational form of heal-ing that was bound to earn the wrath of the doctors and scientists of the Age of Reason. The clinic Mesmer opened was so instantly popular that he took to magnetiz-ing people on a mass-production basis. Even aristocrats, generals, and politicians had to wait their turn to get magnetized.

Mesmer was a showman as well as a healer. Groups of patients in his magnificently appointed consulting rooms would stand in baths of dilute sulphuric acid and iron filings. They joined hands with each other and grasped protruding iron bars. Music and perfume filled the air as Mesmer, wearing a scarlet silk gown, went from patient to patient, touching each with a long metal rod.

"Some patients remain quiet and calm and experience nothing," wrote a member of the Royal Academy of Sciences. "Others cough, spit, feel some slight pain, local heat or general heat, and they perspire. Others are shaken and rocked by convulsions, which are extraordinary by their number, duration, and force. They have been known to persist for more than three hours." Mesmer's assistants would carry the patients experiencing hysterical seizures into an adjoining room, padded on all sides. Such convulsions, comparable to those seen today at the conversion rituals of certain religious sects, were the famous "crises" that led to Mesmer's most impressive cures.

In primitive cultures, of course, it is the medicine man who goes into trance. Behaving as if possessed by a supernatural force, he draws the evil spirits out of the patient. Mesmer turned things around by arranging for the patient, not himself, to go into trance and do battle with the evil spirits.

As the great magnetizer, Mesmer became the rage of Paris, the talk of Europe, and a wealthy man. His success and that of his disciples and imitators posed such a challenge to established medicine that the medical schools began to close down. "In retrospect," Spiegel comments, "that was probably a good thing. The things they were teaching were doing more harm than good." Bloodletting was the standard practice at the time, and undoubtedly many died of it. In contrast, Mesmer was doing much good and little harm.

The controversy about animal magnetism, emotionally debated by Mesmer's admirers and opponents, led, in 1784, to the appointment by Louis XVI of an investigating commission of physicians and scientists. Among the commissioners were the ambassador of the United States, Benjamin Franklin; the great chemist and discoverer of oxygen, Antoine Lavoisier; and a man whose name, like Mesmer's, would become part of the language: Dr. Joseph I. Guillotin.

The commission concluded that animal magnetism was a fake. The convulsions and other "violent effects," said Franklin and his colleagues, "are to be attributed to the touching, to the aroused imagination, and to the mechanical imitation which leads us in spite of ourselves to repeat that which strikes our senses." As we now know, two centuries later, "aroused imagination" is about as good a thumbnail description of the hypnotic state as any. The king added his own opinion, saying that the magnetizer's power could be compared to the emotional attraction that one sex exerts over the other. He anticipated Sigmund Freud, who one day would find in hypnosis the compliance and absence of critical judgment that can be seen in people in love.

Mesmer was discredited. He left Paris and spent the rest of his life in relative obscurity, dying in 1815. Magnetism or mesmerism, however, lived on despite the disapproval of the mandarins of medicine. The plain truth was that this strange and apparently inexplicable mind-arousing technique often provided a remedy that conventional medical practice could not supply.

Among the legions of magnetizers on both sides of the Atlantic was the American physician, Dr. Elisha Perkins, a founding member of the Connecticut Medical Society. In 1795 he discovered that simple pieces of metal, skillfully applied, could draw pain from the body. Soon Perkins was going about the country demonstrating and selling his patented "Tractors." They were metal tongs painted gold and silver that seemed to be able to cure arthritis, rheumatism, and any number of other ailments. George Washington was one of his customers.

Perkins was expelled from the medical society when he refused to defend himself against charges of quackery. He died soon afterward in the 1799 yellow fever epidemic in New York while trying to combat the disease with his Tractors. The controversy in America about tractoration or Perkinism was duplicated in Europe. There, respectable physicians announced that Tractors really did cause pain to disappear, at least with some of their patients. A Perkinean Institute was founded in London. Some enthusiasts predicted that Perkinism would make the family doctor obsolete. The craze quickly subsided, however, after Dr. John Haygarth of Bath disclosed that he had achieved miraculous cures of his own by painting wooden tongs to look like metal and persuading his patients that the instruments, in accordance with Perkins's theory, were draining excess "electroid" from their bodies.

Echoing the conclusions of Benjamin Franklin and others who had investigated Mesmer's work in France, Haygarth declared that both the genuine and fake Tractors produced cures because of the stimulated imagination of the patients. Neither Haygarth nor the vast majority of other men of science were inspired to look more deeply into the apparent self-healing properties of the human mind. According to a study of mesmerism and Perkinism by two Cornell University historians of psychiatry, Eric T. Carlson and Meribeth M. Simpson, "Mesmer and Perkins had drawn in similar fashion on popular theories of physics of their day in order to explain their therapeutic successes, but once the true sources of their cures, imagination and suggestion, became apparent, the whole matter was pushed aside. The powers of suggestion had been dramatically demonstrated, but for legitimate medicine there seemed no way to put this curious weapon to use."

In the mid-1800s, another American, Phineas Parkhurst Quimby of Maine, won fame as a magnetic healer. A blacksmith's son, Quimby had become so adept at mesmerism after witnessing a demonstration by a visiting Frenchman that he abandoned his work as a clockmaker in order to go about New England giving exhibitions of his mind-bending powers. On more than one occasion he was chased out of town by mobs who wanted no part of his "witchcraft." Success came when he devoted himself to healing. Though he believed that he had special magnetic powers, he also was aware that the confidence his patients placed in him had a lot to do with the cures he achieved.

Quimby would be little remembered today were it not for a seemingly miraculous cure that took place one October day in 1862. A forty-one-year-old woman, sensitive and intelligent, had been in delicate health since her birth. When the early death of her first husband was followed by other personal tragedies, she sank into invalidism. According to Sibyl Wilbur, her biographer, "She was afflicted with a spinal weakness which caused spasmodic seizures, followed by prostration which amounted to a complete nervous collapse." Her father would carry her from her bed like a child. Her second husband, a dentist who tried homeopathic treatments, could not make her well. Finally, as "a frail shadow of a woman," she went to see Quimby in his Portland office.

"Gazing fixedly into her eyes," writes Wilbur, "he told her, as he had told others, that she was held in bondage by the opinions of her family and physicians, that her animal spirit was reflecting its grief upon her body and calling it spinal disease. He then wet his hands in a basin of water and violently rubbed her head, declaring that in this manner he imparted healthy electricity. Gradually he wrought the spell of hypnotism, and under that suggestion she let go the burden of pain just as she would have done had morphine been administered. The relief was no doubt tremendous. Her gratitude certainly was unbounded. She felt free from the excruciating pain of years. Quimby himself was amazed at her sudden healing; no less was he amazed at the interpretation she immediately placed upon it, that it had been accomplished by Quimby's mediatorship between herself and God.

"She had come to Quimby prepared to find him a saint who healed by virtue of his religious wisdom, and as soon as she met him she completed her mental picture, endowing him with her own faith. Thus the hypnotist had almost nothing to do. Her faith returned upon her, flooding her with radiance, healing her of her pain."

The patient was Mary Baker Eddy. The cure was permanent. So complete was her transformation from weakness to strength that within four years of her encounter with Quimby, whom she served for a time as the interpreter of his "Science of Health," she founded Christian Science.

There is every reason to believe, as does Dr. Spiegel, that Mrs. Eddy was a highly hypnotizable personality. Her physical ailments seem to have been more hysterical than organic. Wilbur's *The Life of Mary Baker Eddy* tells of "voices" she heard as a child. Her father worried so much about her absorption in books that he ordered them removed, saying, "She must not hear so many exciting tales or be allowed to brood in fancy." She had several profound religious experiences. On February 1, 1866, a month after Quimby's death, she fell on an icy sidewalk and suffered a severe concussion and a spinal dislocation. She was expected to die. God, however, according to her own account, revealed Himself to her and said, "Daughter, arise!" She arose from her bed, dressed, and walked into the parlor where a minister and friends had gathered for a final visit with the dying patient. This was the occasion for her discovery of "Christian Science or divine laws of Life, Truth, and Love."

Though others might see common elements at work in the cures achieved by Christian Scientists and cures that are accomplished by hypnotic techniques, Mrs. Eddy was vehement in denying any connection. Indeed, she denounced hypnotism as an evil and enslaving force. In contrast, she wrote, "the Scientist reaches his patient through divine love." Healing can be accomplished in a single visit "and the disease will vanish into its native nothingness like dew before the morning sunshine."

Despite the widespread American interest in mesmerism and other mind-stimulating ceremonies, it was in Europe that trance phenomena were most seriously investigated. There hypnosis was forged into a medical tool.

Even at the time of the craze over Mesmer's magnetic cures, a more rational understanding of trance behavior was provided by the Marquis de Puységur. In imitation of Mesmer, he magnetized an elm tree—or so he and the peasants in the region believed. A number of the peasants found relief from their sufferings after touching the tree. The marquis was surprised to see that these simple people did not experience hysterical fits while being cured. Apparently Mesmer's sophisticated Parisians went into convulsions because they knew it was the thing to do or because they were imitating the behavior of others.

The most impressive of the cases observed by the marquis was that of a young shepherd who was ailing from an inflammation of the lungs. He would go into a "sleeping trance" yet continue talking as if awake. His behavior was that of a sleepwalker. Afterward, he would have no memory of his actions. While in trance he spoke with extraordinary intelligence about his own disease and with amazing prescience about the troubles of others. "Magnetic somnambulism" was the term given by the marquis to the shepherd's trance state. For decades thereafter, many thought of the mind state produced by magnetism as artificial somnambulism or sleepwalking. As for the youth's insightful intelligence while in trance, that was dubbed "clairvoyance."

Among other experimenters who found that mesmeric theatrics were not necessary for trance-state healing was an abbot named Faria. He came from Goa, the Portuguese enclave in India. Faria performed more than five thousand trance inductions in public by using a simple technique. After gazing fixedly at his subjects, he would instruct them to sit in a chair and close their eyes. Then he would give the loud command, "Sleep!" Ordinary folk in those days would normally be in awe of and submissive to a nobleman, priest, professor, or doctor. A command from an authority figure was something to be obeyed, not questioned. Although Faria supposed that the subject's blood somehow thinned out during the experience, he more accurately insisted that expectation and the impressionability of the subject brought about the trance not magnetism. Above all, he showed how easily and quickly trance could be induced.

At a time when there were few means to combat pain, a number of doctors discovered that they could use this newfangled "induced sleep" to perform painless operations. Although almost all of the leading figures in medicine denounced such activities, the greatest champion of mesmerism in the mid-nineteenth century was one of the most renowned physicians of his time, Dr. John Elliotson, a surgeon, educator, and medical pioneer who is widely credited with introducing the use of the stethoscope in England. The publication in 1837 of a paper describing his employment of mesmerism to perform pain-free surgery touched off such a barrage of criticism from his colleagues that he was forced to resign his professorship at London's University Hospital. Undaunted, he founded a hospital of his own—a "mesmeric hospital" that proved to be the forerunner of similar institutions in the British Isles.

One of Elliotson's admirers was James Esdaile, a Scottish surgeon working in Calcutta. He had read several articles on magnetism and decided to try it on an Indian convict during surgery. When the patient declared that he had felt no pain during the operation and "very little" afterward, Esdaile became a convert to mesmerism. He used it with such success that the governor of Bengal encouraged him to set up a mesmeric hospital. Indian princes as well as peasants flocked to Esdaile's operating rooms. Because of their fear of surgery, many of them had not sought help for such afflictions as scrotal tumors weighing from 10 to 103 pounds. One of the tumors he removed was so big that the patient had used it for a writing desk.

European observers sent home glowing reports of Esdaile's painless cures. They were echoed more than a century later by American visitors to Communist China who told of watching, in the words of Dr. Paul Dudley White, "fully conscious patients undergo major surgery with nothing more than acupuncture and the thoughts of Chairman Mao to comfort them."

All that is necessary for the success of this new and remarkably safe procedure, Esdaile wrote in *Mesmerism in India*, is "passive obedience in the patient and a sustained attention and patience on the part of the operator." His trance inductions—passing his hands up and down the patient's body—varied from two minutes to two hours, but once satisfied that a deep mesmeric "sleep" was under way, he could operate with swift efficiency because of the extraordinary stillness of the patient. On one occasion, he removed a cancerous eye while the other eye looked on unblinkingly. But mesmerism did not work for everyone, as Esdaile freely admitted. Some patients could not or would not go into trance. Some who did enter the trance state showed signs of hurt and anxiety during surgery but not to the degree that would normally be expected. As Esdaile said of one man: "He has only been disturbed by a nightmare, of which on waking he retains no recollection."

During the six years that Esdaile practiced in India, he performed several thousand surgical procedures, including nearly three hundred major operations, with mesmerism as the sole means of stifling pain. He succeeded in reducing the usual postsurgery mortality from 50 percent to 5 percent. When he returned home to Scotland, however, Esdaile found that his mesmeric techniques, while still valuable, did not work quite so well as they did in India. His Scottish patients, he concluded, were more difficult to mesmerize because they were less compliant than Indian patients, whose "nervous fluids" were at a lower ebb. He did not allow for the social and political differences between a skeptical Scot who might respect a physician but not be in awe of him and a typical Indian patient, especially one from a lower caste, who would be obedient and even worshipful in the presence of a medical representative of the ruling British.

Despite the ample evidence of Esdaile's accomplishments in India and the testimony of reputable men who had witnessed his operations, he was denounced by his peers in Britain as a charlatan and a fraud. One physician called his work sacrilegious because he was interfering with God's intention that man should feel pain. Medical journals refused to print his papers. He called himself "the best abused man in the world."

Another Scottish surgeon, James Braid, whose practice was in Manchester, was more fortunate as he risked his reputation by taking an interest in mesmerism.

Doubting the existence of a universal magnetic fluid, Braid established that a person could go into trance merely by gazing at an object—as his own wife did by staring at the lid of a sugar bowl for two and a half minutes. Because Braid viewed trance as "nervous sleep," he coined the word *hypnosis*, drawing on the Greek *hypnos* for sleep. It was an unfortunate choice, as it turns out, for a state of mind that is actually the opposite of sleep.

Noting that the entranced person is exceptionally open to suggestion, Braid attributed the effects of hypnosis to psychological rather than physiological forces. And he concluded that different people go to different levels of trance: from "slight hypnosis" to "deep hypnosis" to the "hypnotic coma."

James Braid has been called the father of modern hypnosis. His scientific approach to trance phenomena made magnetism or mesmerism, now reborn as hypnotism, a more legitimate medical tool. As more and more doctors adopted trance techniques despite the continuing hostility of the medical establishment, it appeared that hypnosis was on its way to being the principal means for providing pain relief in the Western world. But it was not to be. Chemical anesthesia appeared on the scene at the very time of Braid's contributions to enlightenment about the hypnotic trance. Physicians who turned eagerly to nitrous oxide, chloroform, and ether had no time for hypnosis.

Still, there were some who remained fascinated by the uses of trance in medicine. The work of the most important of them paved the way for psychoanalysis. In the Nancy region of France, an obscure country doctor named Ambroise Auguste Liébeault cured many of his poor patients by putting them into trance and bombarding them with suggestions that they would get well, they would be cured, they would be healthy. His work came to the attention of a celebrated physician, Hippolyte Bernheim, a professor at the University of Nancy medical school. One of Bernheim's patients was a man who had suffered from sciatica, a very painful nerve inflammation, for six years. After Bernheim failed to help him during six months of treatment, the patient went to Liébeault and was quickly cured by the country doctor's strange methods.

Setting out to expose Liébeault as a quack, the professor ended up so impressed by what he observed that he became Liébeault's champion as well as a convert to hypnosis himself. In 1886, in his book *Suggestive Therapeutics*, Bernheim described his success in using hypnosis for everything from gastric ailments and aphonia (loss of the capacity to speak) to tremors and sleepwalking. Like Liébeault, he concluded that hypnosis was a state that could be induced in normal persons through suggestion.

This viewpoint of the "Nancy School" of hypnotism came into conflict late in the nineteenth century with the outlook of the "Salpêtrière School," led by the most celebrated neurologist of his day, Jean Martin Charcot. Basing his opinions on the behavior of hysterical patients at the hospital of Salpêtrière in Paris, Charcot came to the conclusion that hypnosis was a pathological condition.

A student of Charcot's, Pierre Janet, while also linking hypnosis and hysteria, put greater stress on psychological instead of neurophysiological changes. The patient in trance *dissociated*, he said, and entered a different order of reality. The idea of hypnosis as dissociation—which many of today's experts believe—was somewhat in line with Bernheim's definition of hypnotism as "the induction of a peculiar psychical condition which increases the susceptibility to suggestion."

In time, the view of the Nancy School about the normality of hynotizable persons would prevail. Hypnosis researchers came to see the error of the Salpétrière School's belief that trance susceptibility amounted to mental disturbance. (Today Spiegel carries things still further by interpreting hypnotic responsivity as a sign of healthy mental functioning.) For a young Viennese physician named Sigmund Freud, it was all very confusing as he embarked on his own hypnotic explorations in the 1880s.

One of Freud's colleagues, Joseph Breuer, had already satisfied himself that the symptoms of hysteria could be removed through hypnotic suggestion. In the now famous case of Anna O., Breuer employed hypnosis to uncover traumatic memories, liberate her repressed emotions, and bring an end to her hysterics. Intrigued by such demonstrations of the value of hypnosis, Freud observed Charcot's work at Salpêtrière and consulted with Liébeault and Bernheim at Nancy. His own use of hypnosis in the following years led directly to his revelations of the importance of the unconscious.

Freud found, however, that hypnosis had its limitations. Not everyone could be hypnotized. And even those who went deeply into trance were able to resist a complete uncovering of repressed emotions. On occasion, hypnosis worked all too well in terms of a patient's readiness to express feelings. Freud was greatly embarrassed one day when, as a servant looked on, he was embraced and kissed by a woman he had hypnotized. All things considered, he thought it best to turn to free association and other techniques that did not require a trance induction.

Although Freud would say in 1918, that, in time, "the pure gold of analysis will be alloyed with such popular methods as hypnosis and suggestions," his decision to abandon hypnosis in his own work led many of his disciples and the legions of analysts who followed them to reject hypnosis altogether. At the same time, the emergence of psychology as an exciting new field of study shifted the attention of scholars away from trance phenomena. Physicians who were using new medicines, instruments, and chemical painkillers had no interest in "unscientific" approaches to healing. To a great extent, hypnosis in the early decades of this century was left to charlatans, stage hypnotists, and dabblers in the occult. A sure way for a doctor to tarnish his professional reputation was to reveal an interest in hypnotism.

Even so, there were a few daring souls who carried on the work of clinical and experimental hypnosis. Clark Hull, a psychologist and authority on learning, did pioneering studies in suggestibility out of his hypnosis laboratory at Yale. Milton Erickson became the country's best known and most controversial medical hypnotist when he devised ingenious trance-state strategies and inspired other therapists to try hypnosis as an aid to treatment.

More often, however, therapeutic hypnosis was employed in other forms, under other labels. At Harvard,

Edmund Jacobson, a physiological psychologist who was an early investigator of the impact of the imagination on the workings of the body, became convinced that muscle tension was the cause of innumerable human ailments. People could find relief, he said, by taking charge of their muscles and discharging the tension. His Progressive Relaxation system, adopted by many medical professionals, was the forerunner by half a century of some of today's popular methods for relaxing and getting in touch with bodily functions.

In Germany, a contemporary of Jacobson's, a neurologist and psychiatrist named J. H. Schultz, was aware of the prejudice against hypnosis in medicine yet impressed by the way patients who used self-hypnosis could relieve their tensions and rid themselves of symptoms. He created Autogenic Training, a complicated series of self-hypnotic exercises involving relaxation, "passive concentration," and imagery. While hugely successful in Europe, his system for self-mastery did not fare so well in the United States. Americans who liked quick results were less willing to devote months of their time to Schultz's long training program.

More to the American taste were the proposals of Emil Coué, a French druggist who found fame in the 1920s with his lectures on "Self-mastery Through Autosuggestion." He propounded the dictum that "Our actions spring, not from our will, but from our imagination." Any number of real or imagined ailments could be cured, he said, if people would only constantly repeat twelve words: "Day by day, in every way, I am getting better and better." Coué set the style for other men who would appear with gospels of self-persuasion, self-improvement, and positive thinking—all of which drew on hypnotic principles and techniques.

Hypnosis, in short, was still very much alive even if in disguise and out of favor with the doctors. It would take World War II to bring hypnosis out of the shadows, give it a secure foothold in medical practice, and show the public its vast potential for summoning the powers of the mind.

5

DISCOVERIES

When a man knows he is to be hanged in a fortnight, it concentrates his mind wonderfully.

—SAMUEL JOHNSON, Boswell's *Life of Johnson*

On December 7, 1941, Dr. Herbert Spiegel of McKeesport, Pennsylvania, was at work at St. Elizabeth's Hospital in Washington, D.C. He had only recently completed his psychiatric residency. As a U.S. Army reservist, he was "on hold": available in case America went to war. The attack on Pearl Harbor that day not only put him in uniform but paved the way for his first encounter with a subject that was considered to be a black sheep of medicine: hypnosis.

By January 1942, First Lieutenant Spiegel was attached to the base hospital at Fort Meade, Maryland. He was also, as an aspiring psychoanalyst, still in analysis. The army allowed him to continue his sessions with Dr. Lewis Hill of Baltimore.

"One day," Spiegel recalls, "I was getting off the couch and Dr. Hill asked me if I'd like to learn about hypnosis. Since this was my analyst, I wondered: What is he trying to say to me? What's the significance of this? Is there some profound statement here? He explained that Adolf

Meyer, who was the chief of psychiatry at Johns Hopkins University, ran a kind of underground railway that had saved hundreds of Jewish and other European intellectuals who were victims of the Nazis. These people were brought to this country in various secret ways and many of them settled in the Baltimore area.

"One of them was Dr. Gustave Aschaffenburg, an elderly man who had been Professor of Forensic Psychiatry at the University of Cologne. He was here as a political refugee. Technically, he was an enemy alien but he wanted to do something, anything, to help win the war. So he passed the word around that he would be glad to teach hypnosis to any army or navy doctors who were interested. My feeling about hypnosis at the time was that it was vaudeville stuff. As a psychiatrist, I took the classical position that Freud had started with hypnosis and then gave it up. I didn't want to bother with it. But my analyst said hypnosis would be useful in my military work, and that got me interested. I began going to the evening sessions that Aschaffenburg held in his Baltimore apartment.

"He was a slight, stooped-over man who spoke in broken English—a typical frail, fragile European intellectual. As a boy he had had chicken pox. An infection of one of the lesions had left him with a very deep and very noticeable scar right in the center of his forehead. Years later, when he was doing a study of criminals at the prison in Cologne, he noticed that a number of them, during his interviews, would gaze at his scar and become so transfixed that they would sort of phase out. Although he was impatient at first with behavior that seemed disrespectful, he realized that something important was happening. The prisoners, instead of paying attention to the interview, focused so much on his scar that they slipped into a different state of consciousness—a trance state. This moved his interest into what he later identified as hypnosis. He began to use it in his psychiatric work."

For Spiegel, this anecdote proved to be important for his understanding of the hypnotic trance because it suggested that hypnosis is something that can occur without a formal ceremony. "It can happen whether anyone decides to do it or not," he says. "Without realizing it or meaning to do it, the prisoners hypnotized themselves by becoming fascinated with the doctor's scar." The scar was the equivalent of the glittering watch or the spot on the wall that a traditional hypnotist might use to induce a trance.

Not long after beginning his studies with Aschaffenburg, Spiegel was able to put his knowledge of hypnosis to good use at Fort Meade. At three o'clock one morning, while he was serving as officer-of-the-day at the hospital, the military police brought in a dazed and totally confused young woman who had been found wandering around the outskirts of the post. She said she didn't know her name or where she had come from.

"I remembered what Aschaffenburg had told us about hysterical amnesia. It is clear now that someone with hysterical amnesia is almost sure to be highly hypnotizable but I was not aware of it then. So I took a deep breath and asked her to fix her eyes on something. To my absolute astonishment, she immediately went into a profound trance state. I was almost frightened when I saw it. And then she abreacted: She had this great emotional release of her tensions and the whole story just poured out.

"We learned that she was the wife of a sergeant on the base. Someone had sent her a letter saying that her husband was involved in hanky-panky with girls around the post. So without thinking much about it, she hopped on a bus. Then as she approached the camp she realized that there was going to be a confrontation and she might find out some things she didn't want to find out. Her conflict was so intense that she just divorced herself from her identity as a protection against the impending crisis. She disconnected from her own awareness. I was able to use the trance both to get information about her and to help her restore some of her former self-regard. In the meantime, the chaplain brought her husband to the hospital and did some instant marital counseling. They were soon embracing and making up. The crisis was over. I had a lot of respect for the trance state after that."

One other incident at Fort Meade "is not something I'm proud of," Spiegel admits, but he relates it to the doctors at his hypnosis courses as an example of how *not* to use hypnosis in therapy.

A young black infantryman arrived at the station hospital with a paralyzed left arm. Since it appeared to be a case of hysterical paralysis, Spiegel guided him into a trance and with a few well-chosen words quickly removed the symptom. The man could move his arm with normal ease. The paralysis would return, however, each time that Spiegel touched the man's back. The soldier was unaware that the doctor had planted a posthypnotic signal during the trance state. (A highly hypnotizable person, as this soldier appears to have been, may respond to a signal outside trance, because of instructions given while in trance, and yet be unable to account for his reaction because he had also been told to forget that an instruction had been given.)

Physicians and other officers, including the commander of the hospital, came around to witness the use of hypnosis to turn a paralysis on and off. After repeating the demonstration several times, Spiegel realized that he was treating the enlisted man like a performer in a show. Difficult as it was to give up such a good subject, he sent his patient back to duty. Three days later, the soldier returned to the hospital with both arms and both legs paralyzed. Spiegel suspected that the paralysis had come back stronger than ever because of the inappropriate and undignified way in which the man had been treated.

"This time," he says, "I dealt with him as a person instead of as an amusing object." The soldier was hypnotized once again. The paralysis was removed. Seeking the cause of the problem, Spiegel learned that the soldier was having difficulty with a white sergeant who seemed to be against him. Because he wanted to fight back but knew he shouldn't, his body produced its own answer to the dilemma. His "paralyzed" arm prevented him from striking the sergeant. Having apologized for the earlier treatment, Spiegel arranged to have the soldier assigned to a more agreeable unit to prevent a recurrence of the problem. The man was still doing well when inquiries were made six months later.

By that time, the summer of 1942, Spiegel himself was on his way to new duties. He had received secret orders to report to the First Infantry Division. Arriving at Indiantown Gap, Pennsylvania, and garbed in his summer uniform, he suspected that he was about to go overseas when he saw that everyone else was wearing winter clothing.

"They impounded my car because everything was so secret," he remembers. "We were due to sail the next day on the *Queen Elizabeth*. I wasn't even allowed to call my family to say good-bye. I learned that I was the last-minute replacement for some medical officer who had conveniently gotten sick just before shipping out. When I reported to headquarters, they asked me, 'Lieutenant Spiegel, are you a surgeon?' I said, 'No, I'm a psychiatrist.' You should have heard them laugh. What a joke! 'All right,' they said, 'you're an M.D. but have you ever had any field experience?' I told them the closest I'd come was Boy Scout training. Another big joke! Then they asked, 'Is your will made out?' When I said I had no will, they threw a form at me and told me to make one out. I was told that I was now an assistant battalion surgeon. All military doctors are called surgeons. I had been pulled out of psychiatry because I was young and healthy, but it all happened so fast that I missed the special course on combat medicine for doctors. I knew nothing about basic infantry tactics, setting up an aid station, and so on. I said, 'How will I know what to do?' They said, 'Just follow us, doc.' "

Spiegel's parents had not expected him to become a doctor. His father had emigrated to the United States from Austria-Hungary soon after the turn of the century and, years later, had started a food-distribution business in McKeesport, Pennsylvania, with his brother and a third partner. His mother was the daughter of a Pennsylvania dairy farmer who had also come over from Austria-Hungary. Herbert, born in 1914, was expected to go into the family firm. Soon after graduating from high school, however, and after being accepted at a leading business college, he decided to go in another direction.

"It dawned on me," he explains, "that I really didn't want to spend the rest of my life in wholesale groceries." He was influenced by a relative who was a pathologist and by a Boy Scout leader who became a physician. Spiegel attended college and medical school at the University of Maryland. After receiving his M.D. in 1939, he went on to St. Francis Hospital in Pittsburgh for a year of general internship and to St. Elizabeth's for his psychiatric residency. Now, in the summer of 1942, he was aboard the world's largest ship, a ship bursting at the seams with fifteen thousand American infantrymen as it zigzagged to Scotland without an escort in four and a half days.

After several months of training and waiting in

Scotland and England, the First Infantry Division was crammed into a motley collection of vessels that joined the rest of the 650 ships of Operation Torch, soon to be acclaimed in the press as "the greatest amphibious invasion in history." The combined American and British forces, 157,000 strong, landed at Casablanca, Oran, and Algiers on November 8, 1942. "Since our ship, an old mail steamer, had kept its civilian crew," Spiegel recalls, "officers like myself would be awakened each morning by the steward in his white jacket serving coffee. On the morning of the invasion he knocked at the door at four o'clock and served us coffee. Then we put on our battle gear, scrambled down the nets, and went to war."

Operation Torch, directed by General Eisenhower from Gibraltar, was intended to clear North Africa of Rommel's desert army in preparation for the assault on the supposedly soft underbelly of Europe. The job was expected to take six weeks. In fact, six months were required to force the German surrender of May 13, 1943. Spiegel was in the thick of a nightmare operation that hurled green American troops led by untested officers against battle-hardened Germans.

As a psychiatrist, he was supposed to be tending the mentally afflicted in a U.S. hospital, not patching up bodies under fire in Africa. His mood was not improved by the knowledge that he was a lieutenant doing a captain's job. The suddenness of his assignment to the division had caused the foul-up. "And besides all that," he says, "you can get hurt out there." But it was also the opportunity of a lifetime and an experience that shaped his career. "I was taken out of my specialty yet I learned more about psychiatry, people, and my own ability to deal with a crisis than in any other year in my life." As compensation for great risk, he was granted the kind of firsthand observation of human reactions to the maximum stress of a battlefield that few of his colleagues in psychiatry would ever know.

Overconfident after quickly subduing the Vichy French forces in Morocco and Algeria, the American troops rolled into Tunisia and were caught in horrendous battles in that bleak and barren country. Morale was poor. Too often they were sent the wrong ammunition or were hit by their own aircraft. More than 2,400 U.S. soldiers were taken prisoner when the Germans triumphed at the Kasserine Pass. Nazi propagandists told the world about panicking American GIs. Eisenhower rushed in General Patton to get things shaped up, which he did, but Spiegel's outfit came close to being wiped out when it was trapped in a valley just before the epic tank battle at El Guettar. The American victory in that duel, however, marked the beginning of the great push that forced the surrender of nearly a quarter million Germans and cleared the way for the landings in Sicily.

Under such conditions, doctoring becomes as basic as it can possibly be. In contrast to the usual priorities of an emergency room, combat imperatives demand that the first patients to be treated are those with the least critical wounds so that they can be rushed back into action. The gravely wounded must take their chances. A battalion surgeon has to improvise, improve on the rule book, and do whatever works best in the circumstances. It is hardly surprising, given this unconventional start in psychiatry, that Spiegel became a most unconventional practitioner in civilian life.

Psychotherapy under fire is bound to be rough and ready. Spiegel remembers at El Guettar "being hit so hard from all directions, including Stuka dive-bomber attacks, that we were stuck. We couldn't go forward or backward. Suddenly my jeep driver started running around, crying, 'I can't take it! I can't take it.' He begged me to send him to the rear. I grabbed him by the shirt and told him, 'You no good son of a bitch, the only way you'll get out of here is when your body is carried out! You're staying with us! Now go dig yourself a hole and stay in it until I tell you when to get out!'

"So he dug a foxhole so deep he could have had a guest in there with him. Several hours later, when things had calmed down, I went over to him and we talked. He said he felt better. He was able to continue in combat for the rest of the North African campaign. Then, in the landing in Sicily, he was wounded. It was a minor wound so they made him a hospital orderly. For years after the war he sent me Christmas cards thanking me for helping him get over his fright and keep his wits together. A lot of other soldiers who panicked like that were carelessly evacuated as nut cases and ended up with a great sense of guilt, not thinking of themselves as real men, because they had 'chickened out' and left their buddies to do the fighting."

Spiegel was wounded himself on the last day of the Tunisian campaign. A shell fragment, so hot that it seared the boot as it drove through, tore into his right ankle and broke the lower tibia. He felt a general pain but did not know where he had been struck until he saw a piece of steel stuck in his leg like an arrowhead. He did not realize that he burned his hand pulling it out until later when he noticed the blisters. Thinking that he was probably hit elsewhere if his pain was general rather than specific, he asked an aide to examine him. There was nothing else. The realization that he had only a single "dream wound"—bad enough to get away from the front lines but not so bad that he would be disfigured or disabled—gave him such a feeling of elation that he did not need a painkiller during the jarring four-mile ride on a litter to the mobile hospital.

The pain was there, all right. He had to hold up his leg

to minimize it. Yet his *perception* of the pain was such that it seemed agreeable and welcome in light of his escape from death or a terrible mutilation. Years later, when teaching doctors about hypnosis, he would be able to call on this memory as he explained how a patient, in trance, can "filter the hurt out of the pain."

Spiegel's battalion commander gave him a battlefield promotion to captain before sending him to the rear. He was shipped home in June 1943 after nearly a year overseas. Several weeks passed, however, before the army chiefs realized that a psychiatrist who mistakenly had been sent into combat was now at hand and no doubt full of information and insights about battlefront conditions. When interviewed by a series of generals and other officers, he had some scathing things to say about policies and practices that worked against troop morale. "My main impression," he recalls, "was that these people who were running the war really didn't know what was going on in the field. I never had nightmares during combat, but after those interviews in Washington I had battle dreams for the first time."

Spiegel remained in uniform for four and a half years, until the spring of 1946, though not because of any fondness for the military. He was anxious to return to civilian life, but his specialty was in ever greater demand as the number of Americans in combat around the world increased and as the psychiatric casualties mounted. Most of his time was spent at the School of Military Neuropsychiatry at Mason General Hospital (now Pilgrim State Hospital) on Long Island, New York, treating the mentally wounded and training civilian psychiatrists for military work. Mason General was the largest army psychiatric facility in the world, collecting patients from all theaters of war. On occasion, Spiegel remembers, two hospital ships would arrive in New York at the same time and as many as a thousand casualties would have to be processed at the hospital in a single day.

Such wartime pressures led to the resurrection of hypnosis as a psychiatric tool. Many soldiers were disabled because of traumatic experiences during combat. While blocking out the memory of a terrible event, a GI might express his reaction to the horror through the body metaphor of a paralysis, loss of speech, blindness, or another symptom. The strategy of the doctors was to reach into the mind, uncover the event, and encourage an abreaction, or emotional discharge. Psychoanalysis was one approach, but there were too many patients and too little time. Hypnosis was the best shortcut. A soldier in trance could be helped to remember the origins of his illness. If he happened to be highly hypnotizable and thus capable of age regression, he could virtually relive the traumatic experience.

"The big issue," Spiegel comments, "is that the memory of the event becomes fused with the horror of the event. Every time you remember what happened, you get the horror again. And so you develop an amnesia in order to avoid the horror. The point of therapy is to separate the memory from the horror so that it can be remembered without an emotional outburst—just as we can mourn the loss of a loved one without repeating our reactions at the time of death. You want the memory to become part of your historical past instead of your hysterical present.

"It's better for the patient to get these things out in the open. Freud postulated that the more we abreact to repressed memories, the freer we are in the long run. It's the repressed memories that tend to stir up all kinds of distortions of our present perception. Our whole theory in treating war neuroses was to get the abreaction as exhaustively and completely as possible. Our regret was that we couldn't spend more time with the soldiers."

Spiegel's firsthand experience with both combat conditions and the treatment of mentally disturbed soldiers came to the attention of a distinguished psychoanalyst, Dr. Abram Kardiner, who, until his death in 1981, was one of the oldest living analysands of Sigmund Freud. Kardiner, thirty years Spiegel's senior, invited him to collaborate on an updated version of his book, *War Stress and Neurotic Illness*, which he had written years before after studying the hospital records of World War I survivors. The new work, by Kardiner and Spiegel, was published in 1947.

While working at Mason General, Spiegel, now an army major, was able to make regular journeys into New York City for analytic training at the William Alanson White Institute of Psychiatry. It was a program of study that would go on for six years.

The White Institute was the right place for him. His wartime psychiatric work had already led him to question the value of orthodox analysis in cases that seemed suitable for more direct psychotherapy. Freud's greatness, he felt, was undeniable, but too many of his disciples took every utterance of the master as gospel. "What had started off as a scientific approach to studying behavior had become a kind of religious belief. Fortunately, the White Institute did not have that religious fervor. We were part of the protestant group in the analytic movement. We thought of ourselves as the free thinkers."

Two of his supervisors at the institute, Harry Stack Sullivan and Erich Fromm, were among the more celebrated and innovative thinkers in psychiatry. Known as "neo-analysts" because of their departure from Freud's teachings, they had a strong influence on Spiegel. He notes that

Sullivan, "who did not insist that his patients lie down on a couch," was the first important figure among American psychoanalysts who did not go off to Europe for training. "He wasn't afraid to go his own way." Spiegel's primary supervisor, Frieda Fromm-Reichmann, and his new analyst, Clara Thompson, were instrumental in encouraging him to carry on his interest in hypnosis.

Spiegel has a vivid memory of the day that a noted psychologist and analyst who was using hypnosis at the Menninger Clinic traveled to Mason General to see his work. "She was impressed but when she heard that I was getting training for analysis she gave me a warning. 'If you are serious about analysis,' she said, 'don't let people identify you with hypnosis because it could tarnish your reputation.' She said her own policy at Menninger was to do her work very quietly so that no one thought of her as a hypnotist."

Taking this advice from a senior figure in psychoanalysis very seriously, he mentioned to Clara Thompson that he was thinking of giving up hypnosis. "The next thing I knew, Frieda Fromm-Reichmann called me in and bawled the hell out of me. She wondered what kind of fragile ego I had if I was so concerned about the opinions of other people. We spent the entire session taking apart my ego. She really made me feel like a jerk, so obviously I didn't give up hypnosis."

Fromm-Reichmann went further and arranged to have Spiegel, although only a trainee at the institute, give a series of seminars on hypnosis. She signed up as the first of his students.

The give-and-take of those seminars had a profound impact on Spiegel. They ignited an interest in variations of hypnotic capacity that would lead to the creation of the Hypnotic Induction Profile. Why were some people trance prone and others not? Why did some go deeply into trance and others only so far and no further? What were their personality traits?

Like so many of his associates, Spiegel was still burdened by the excess baggage of hypnosis: the old myths, the hackneyed procedures, the imprecise or misleading terminology. He assumed, as did most psychiatrists, that the hypnotic trance was a sign of hysteria. A person who responded to trance suggestions was commonly described as being "susceptible" to hypnosis, and susceptibility was viewed as an indicator of emotional stress and illness. To be hypnotizable was to be psychologically weak.

"Frieda challenged this notion," Spiegel relates. "She felt that although hypnotizability was identified in stressed persons, it could also be identified in secure, trusting, nonstressed, mentally healthy persons as well. She suggested that I expand my data base to explore this proposal. At first I dismissed this notion. After all, she admitted that she herself did not use hypnosis, whereas I did. But as my work continued, I did indeed learn that not only were secure and healthy people hypnotizable, but the severely mentally ill were not hypnotizable at all."

6

INVESTIGATIONS

It is a wise hypnotist who realizes who is hypnotizing whom.

—HIPPOLYTE BERNHEIM

"Almost any idiot can learn how to hypnotize another
person," Dr. Spiegel says. "Since practically all hypnosis is
self-hypnosis, the idea of my hypnotizing you is just a
ceremonial term. Actually, what you are doing is dis-
covering your trance capacity in response to my proposal
that you go into trance."

His realization that the credit for hypnosis should go
more to the subject than to the hypnotist stems from an
incident, early in his career, involving a soldier who was
under treatment for a mental breakdown during combat.
Spiegel had been invited to demonstrate the Pentothal
interview technique to a group of doctors. While preparing to insert the syringe into the soldier's forearm, he
gave a running commentary on the procedure. "Before
the needle got into the vein, however," he recalls, "and
without receiving one drop of the drug, the soldier went
into a deep trance state. He spontaneously reoriented
himself to the battle experience and went through an intense emotional acting out, with detailed recall, of the

traumatic events that had caused his breakdown. He remained in the trance until he was given the signal to open his eyes. He came out of it with a great sense of relief and he commented about how helpful the medicine was. He said he wished he had received this treatment sooner."

Hypnosis, in short, had happened without any attempt to hypnotize. The patient, not the doctor, was the master of the ceremony. What occurred was as good as hypnosis without being called hypnosis. This was just one of a number of incidents that led Spiegel to think of hypnosis as a setting for the patient's discovery or exercise of his trance capacity. As he told a meeting of the Academy of Psychoanalysis in 1958, this view of hypnosis "represents a reversal of the original concept that the hypnotist projects some mysterious force onto the subject. Instead, it is the hypnotist who structures an occasion for the subject to activate a capacity already developed within himself."

Spiegel had begun questioning much of the conventional wisdom about hypnosis, particularly the notion that it is a form of sleep, soon after his sessions with Dr. Aschaffenburg. He had to discover for himself that misleading ideas about hypnosis are conveyed by the outward appearance of the active, controlling hypnotist and the passive, submissive subject. Few people understood that the subject's compliant and sleeplike condition was just a front for an extraordinarily alert and active engagement of seldom used mental resources. Spiegel's wartime years at Mason General gave him an exceptional opportunity, between therapy and teaching, to carry out investigations of hypnotic phenomena.

In the course of one of his studies, he conducted trance inductions with sixteen of the twenty GIs in a ward. He used a white card with a black dot in the center to focus their attention. A soldier who had not been selected for the study became fascinated by what his buddies had to say about hypnosis. He appeared in Spiegel's office one day, stood at attention, and declared, "Sir, you couldn't hypnotize me even if you wanted to!"

As the soldier was saying this, Spiegel noticed that he was staring at the white card on the desk and that his right eye had closed.

"In that case," Spiegel asked him, "why is your right eye closed?"

"I don't know," the soldier replied, "but my left eye is still open."

"All right," he was told, "now both your eyes will close." The soldier closed his left eye and went into trance.

Spiegel would find that such behavior is not unusual: "People capable of deep trance experiences can manage to get themselves into trance states if the hypnotist does not interfere with the process." He also learned that "the conscious statement doesn't make a bit of difference. It is the unconscious perception that counts. Here was a soldier who really wanted to be in the group. He didn't want to be left out of things and miss the experience. Yet he insisted that he could not be hypnotized."

On another occasion, Spiegel performed a fast and unorthodox hypnotic induction in order to save himself and an enraged soldier from injury.

Responding to a message from the military police that there was a GI in the emergency room who was threatening to kill him, Spiegel went there and was directed to a room where the man had been isolated. As he opened the door and stepped inside the soldier leaped at him, grabbed his throat, and started to choke him. Spiegel was able to wrestle his assailant to the top of a desk. Seeing that the man's face was close to an ink bottle, he held him tightly in position and commanded: "Look at that ink bottle and keep looking at it!'' Immediately, he could feel the soldier's tense muscles relax. He watched in amazement as the man became limp and collapsed to the floor.

The incident was an eye-opener for Spiegel because it demonstrated that highly trance-prone people can be frightened into hypnosis. In the midst of an emotionally charged situation, as he was being overpowered physically, the young soldier had heard the officer-doctor, the voice of authority, give a command to focus all his attention on one thing: the ink bottle. His rage had vanished as he concentrated totally on something else.

Spiegel recognized him as a patient he had seen the week before. Instead of the medical discharge that had been promised him, the soldier had been reassigned to active duty because of a clerical error. And so he took out his anger on his doctor. Spiegel had him readmitted to the hospital for further treatment. No longer hostile, the patient willingly took part in the hypnosis research program that the doctor was conducting.

Although regretting that he had to bully the soldier into a trance, ''because this is not the way a reputable physician using hypnosis treats his patients,'' Spiegel tells the story to make a point about coercion. In intimidating or coercive settings, such as a police interrogation room or a courtroom, authority figures—cops, judges, prosecutors, defense attorneys—may well evoke a trance from a highly hypnotizable individual and not even realize that they have done so. That person, suspending his customary critical judgment while in hypnosis, might go along with suggestions, pick up cues, and end up as an ''honest liar'' as he identifies a suspect or gives an account of a crime. ''The subject confuses the hypnotic implantations with his own knowledge,'' Spiegel explains, ''and by so fusing them, he cannot tell one from the other.''

A crime suspect who is inclined to spontaneous trance states might well confess to a murder—whether guilty or innocent—and afterward have no memory of doing so. For this among other reasons, many experts in clinical and experimental hypnosis oppose the teaching of hypnosis to police officers who wish to use it as an investigative tool. Spiegel argues, however, that it is better to educate police and other legal professionals about hypnosis so that they can identify spontaneous trance states when they occur and avoid creating a hypnotic atmosphere when questioning a witness, victim, or suspect. A confession, in any event, should be considered reliable only if it is buttressed by evidence.

Similarly, because of the possibility of confabulation (the subject replacing fact with fancy) or memory contamination by clumsy questioning, information gleaned by using hypnosis to enhance the recall of crime victims or witnesses should be regarded primarily as leads for more conventional evidence gathering.

The extreme suggestibility of highly hypnotizable individuals in trance is demonstrated by Spiegel in a film, *Fact or Fiction: An Experiment in Post-Hypnotic Compliance*, that was made in 1968 by NBC for possible use in a documentary. It has been shown numerous times at medical and psychological conferences as well as the Columbia hypnosis course.

The volunteer for the experiment was an antiques expert named Charles Snyder who had sought Spiegel's help some time earlier because of the blinding headaches that had plagued him most of his life. His headaches had vanished for good when he learned that he had an exceptional gift for trance. This gave him the means to establish permanent control over his affliction. The experiment took place in an NBC studio in Manhattan. After leading Snyder into the trance state, Spiegel told him that there was a Communist plot under way to seize control of all the major radio and television networks and asserted that this is *"your* important information." Snyder was instructed to "hold firmly to this knowledge and conviction" no matter how strenuously others questioned him about the matter. "If you are pressed hard enough, you will even provide them with facts and figures, and name specific persons to prove your point." He was to stick to his story "whether in or out of the trance, this time or the next time. However, at some later time, when I touch your left shoulder, you will burst into laughter and acknowledge this to be a big joke done as an experiment in human behavior."

When Snyder was brought out of the formal trance by Spiegel and vigorously questioned by the late Frank McGee of NBC News, he insisted that a Communist plot was in progress. Over the course of a long and heated argument, with McGee accusing him of inventing the whole thing and demanding proof, Snyder stuck to his guns and provided details about the conspirators and their plans. He had gotten his information, he declared, from an informant during a beer party in a loft over an Off-Broadway theater "right off Sheridan Square" in Greenwich Village. When the trance state was reinstated and Snyder was again questioned, he held firmly to his story and impassionedly spoke of the need to capture a man named Harris, "the spearhead of the group." He said, "I feel so strongly about it that it makes me tremble to think what might happen in this country."

Snyder laughed when Spiegel touched his left shoulder. He said good-naturedly that he knew some tricks had been played on him but he had no memory of what had occurred. Some months later, when shown the film of the exercise, he was flabbergasted. He was not a beer drinker; he had never been in a Greenwich Village loft; he knew

no one named Harris; and his left-of-center political beliefs made him doubtful of Communist-conspiracy theories. "I just can't conceive of having said the things I
said," Snyder commented. "I don't think that way or believe that way."

Nothing intrigued Spiegel so much during his years as a
military psychiatrist as the phenomenon of age regression. While hypnotizable people can use the trance state
to remember past events more vividly, perhaps even recovering long-forgotten or suppressed details, only a relative few can all but relive earlier times in their lives. They
are the Fives on Spiegel's scale of hypnotizability.

But if an adult is hypnotically regressed to his sixth
birthday and speaks in the present tense in the manner of
a six-year-old, is this a genuine reexperiencing of an earlier time? Or is it the adult's clever attempt, in his desire
to please or fool the hypnotist, to act the part of a child?

What Spiegel was looking for in his research was
"a more controlled and dynamic approach to hypnotic
regression phenomena." As he reported in 1944 to the
annual meeting of the American Psychopathological Association, he developed a "hypnotic ablation technique"
that tested the genuineness of a patient's responses when
regressed to a specified age. "Ablation" seemed to him the
best word to use to describe the temporary removal from
awareness of all information and experiences acquired
after a stated age level. It was like an amputation of memory. A fifty-year-old who reverted to the state of mind of
his fifth year of life, for example, would have no access to
the data or abilities gathered in the succeeding four and a
half decades.

Spiegel would tell a twenty-four-year-old soldier in
trance: "This is no longer the present time. You are going

back into the years. You are getting younger and younger. You're twenty-four years old . . . twenty-three . . . twenty-one . . . nineteen . . . sixteen . . . ten . . . eight . . . seven years old. Today is your seventh birthday. When I touch the side of your head you will be able to open your eyes. You will meet a friend whom you have never seen before. His name is George. He will have something interesting to show you. All right, now you can open your eyes."

By suggesting a specific birthday but avoiding any other suggestion that might interfere with the patient's orientation to a childhood time, Spiegel sought to place him in a particular day in his personal history and let his reactions and observations be entirely spontaneous. Mindful that the patient would have developed some feelings about him (perhaps seeing him as a substitute parent), Spiegel, instead of asking questions himself, would introduce a "friend," a neutral figure, to ask the questions. This associate of Spiegel would begin a conversation with the seven-year-old, ask a few questions ("How old are you? Anything special going on today?"), and then administer one of the major psychological tests for intelligence, performance, vocabulary, and so on. Afterward, Spiegel would step in and touch the patient's forehead and bring him forward through the years to the present.

The test results persuaded Spiegel that the regressed states were "authentic early experiences, somehow recaptured, reawakened, or released, through the hypnotic ablation procedure." Anyone not in trance who tried to simulate psychological functioning at earlier age levels could be detected. As he and his associates wrote at the time in *Psychosomatic Medicine*, the regressed individual "makes efforts to respond and to perform to the best of his ability, utilizing only the learning and growth which had been available to him at that time. He appears to have no access to memories, experiences, and capacities which he had acquired in life later than the suggested age levels."

Later in his career, when he conducted age regressions in the famous case of "Sybil," whose sixteen personalities (or variations of a single highly imaginative personality) made her the subject of a book and motion picture, Spiegel was surprised to find that guiding her back to her childhood birthdays was ineffective. It was like turning to a blank page. But when he asked her about Christmas day when she was ten years old, she reexperienced events of that day with childlike animation. He learned afterward that Sybil's birthdays had not been celebrated because of her family's religious beliefs.

To Spiegel, Sybil was "a brilliant hysteric" with a runaway imagination. When her case was discussed during the trial of a man who claimed not to be responsible for three murders because of his supposed dual personality, Spiegel, as an expert witness, was asked how he could tell whether Sybil's responses in age regression were genuine or whether she was just being a clever actress. "On that Christmas day of the tenth year," he replied, "we had a psychologist come in and give her an intelligence test. She came out with all the answers that were typical of a ten-year-old. We did pycholinguistic tests on her and her speech was typical of a ten-year-old. Then we shifted her to one month old and she didn't talk. She had reflexes like the rooting reflex where, if you touched the side of her face, her head would move. If you put your finger in her hand, she would have a clasp reflex just as an infant would. We put a lit match in front of her and she didn't respond at all. When we lit a match in front of her at the age of six, she said, 'Oh, that's naughty! You're not allowed to touch that!' "

One of Spiegel's patients during his army days was a

sergeant who had gone mad during a battle. As an observer for his artillery unit, he had made some miscalculations about the distance of the enemy. He saw the shell land on his fellow soldiers, including good friends. Psychotic and useless because of this horror, he was shipped back to the United States. He stuttered so badly that he was thought to be a catatonic mute.

"In those days," Spiegel says, "we didn't have the eye roll or Profile but I can say in retrospect that he was a Five. I was able to hypnotize him and use age regression. He had been stuttering terribly but when I regressed him to the day before the incident when he blew his top, he spoke fluently. No stutter at all. Then I regressed him to the year before, and to age twenty, to seventeen, and so on to the first grade of school. No stutter. But when we went to his fifth birthday he started stuttering again. This was really strange! Then when we moved him to his sixth birthday once again, in grade school, he didn't stutter. So we went back to five and then to four, and he stuttered each time.

"When I brought him back to the present, he had no memory of ever stuttering as a kid. We sent a Red Cross social worker to interview his mother. It was a routine social service interview without indicating what we were trying to discover. She learned that the mother used to worry about him as a child because he stuttered. His speech had straightened out, however, as soon as he started going to school. And he had never stuttered since then—until the combat tragedy. This seemed to me a rather pure case of hypnotic age regression serving to get at the truth."

Another soldier, a twenty-five-year-old with comparable trance talent, was easily regressed to earlier age levels but he seemed confused when asked his name on his twelfth birthday. He just looked around and said, "Vass?"

Spiegel realized that the soldier, now speaking as a young-ster, could not understand English. He found someone who spoke German and used him as an interpreter. The twelve-year-old was obviously relieved and readily an-swered questions in fluent German. Spiegel found that he had to use the interpreter for every age level up to and including his thirteenth year. After that, English would do.

"When I brought him out of the trance, I asked him about his personal history. It seems that his family had been compelled to leave Austria when he was thirteen years old. He came to the United States and started to speak English. He had learned to despise German so much that there was no trace of it in his speech as a twenty-five-year-old. Under hypnotic regression, even his handwriting reverted to German script at any age under thirteen. And from thirteen to eighteen his spoken En-glish revealed a gradually disappearing German accent."

Spiegel continued his exploration of hypnotic phenom-ena after leaving the service and going into private prac-tice. By the 1960s, his years of clinical and experimental work had led him to construct three basic principles about hypnosis.

First, *alterations of awareness occur almost constantly*. In addition to the sleep-awake rhythms, there are fre-quent variations in shifts of attention from peripheral to central awareness, from scanning to concentration on one focal area to various fragmented experiences. As he wrote in *The International Journal of Clinical and Ex-perimental Hypnosis*, "Poets, writers, philosophers, clini-cians, and scientists have for centuries alluded to the various levels of awareness that man experiences from day to day, and even from moment to moment. When, under appropriate conditions, the clinician structures an occasion for a shift of awareness to a specific type of dissociation, and enables the patient to remain frozen in that state, we can by definition call this 'hypnosis' even though the only difference between this and other dissociated states that the same patient has experienced is that, in this instance, the patient responds to a stimulus that has been knowingly established and perpetuated by deliberate design for a designated goal.

"This latter feature, the instigation and controlled perpetuation by deliberate design, allows us to label the event with the name 'hypnosis.' It is difficult to estimate the varied number of instances, though, when this occurs without benefit of this 'official' label."

He observed that women who removed the pain of childbirth by using muscle relaxation techniques instead of chemical anesthesia "are most certainly experiencing the equivalent of hypnoanesthesia, even though neither the doctor nor the patient acknowledges, that hypnosis is being used."

Spiegel's second principle was that *hypnotic phenomena occur whether they are identified as such or not.* The soldier who had gone into trance before receiving the Pentothal injection had made this plain to him. So had other patients. He had a special memory of a forty-five-year-old woman whose problem was not only embarrassing but debilitating. She had hiccups that just wouldn't stop.

The patient had been hiccupping constantly for eight days in the wake of a five-month period of indigestion and frequent spasms of air swallowing (aerophagia). The hiccupping was so severe that she was almost incapable of eating or retaining food and fluids. After losing a great deal of weight she was taken to the intensive-care unit at Doctors Hospital in New York and fed intravenously. No method or medication could stop the hiccups. Her internist, with apologies to the woman's husband for resorting to such an unorthodox measure, decided to give hypnosis a try. He asked Dr. Spiegel to see her.

For Spiegel, one vital piece of information was the fact that the woman's hiccups persisted while awake yet stopped when she succeeded in falling asleep. He led her into the trance state and helped her to discover that she could, by relaxing and breathing differently, control the hiccups. She then found that she could do so out of trance. The hiccupping ceased altogether within an hour of Spiegel's arrival. That evening, at precisely ten o'clock, in response to a posthypnotic signal he had given her, she fell into a deep, relaxing sleep. The next day she was removed from the critical list and allowed to go home. There were no more hiccups.

What most interested Spiegel about this case was the fact that the patient had suffered a similar bout of hiccups fifteen years earlier and had been cured in circumstances that could be described as hypnotic. At that time, the woman's prolonged hiccupping had come in the wake of two disk operations to relieve back pain. She was unable to conquer the hiccups until the day her family doctor, after a heart attack, called her to his bedside. He announced that she was his last patient before he went off to retirement in Florida and told her how to carry out a set of breathing instructions.

When Spiegel telephoned the retired physician for details about this episode and suggested that the equivalent of hypnosis had occurred, the man was insulted. "He told me that he did not believe in quack magic. He said he would sue me if I ever told anyone that what he did was hypnosis. He was totally unaware that the emotionally charged situation, the dramatic setting, and his instructions to a patient who was well above average in hypnotizability all amounted to a kind of trance induction. My own encounter with this woman was labeled hypnosis because I *knowingly* elicited the trance state, maintained a sensitive contact with the patient during the trance, and gave her a clear cutoff signal to come out of the trance state. The earlier situation was natural hypnosis, or hypnosis without the label. It merely lacked the formality of someone starting it, maintaining contact, and cutting it off."

In his teachings, Spiegel has asked this question: "Is there any physician in any specialty who has not in the course of years of practice had many occasions to reflect upon the impressive therapeutic response in some patients that could not be understood in terms of the medication administered or the surgical procedure performed? I suspect that quite often the unidentified hypnotic effect was a factor."

Spiegel's third basic principle was this: *Nothing can be achieved in therapy with hypnosis that cannot also be achieved without hypnosis—except that in some instances hypnosis appreciably facilitates the time factor.*

He would cite as an example the case of a thirty-seven-year-old woman who was rushed to the hospital in a comatose condition after swallowing an excessive dosage of barbiturates in an effort to relieve her pain. "I first saw her in the intensive-care unit, where she was receiving continuous intravenous fluids. By this time she had recovered from the immediate toxic effects of the barbiturates and was complaining of severe pain in the left leg, chest pain, nausea, and restlessness. Because of the nausea she was not able to retain any liquids or food. Following a hysterectomy a few years before, she had developed a thrombophlebitis in her left leg, with three episodes of pulmonary embolism. She had recovered each time but was in constant fear of another occurrence."

In short, the patient was in such a bad way that an extended period of treatment in the hospital appeared to be necessary. She was able, however, to go into trance under Spiegel's guidance and learn how to counter the pain with a protective mask of numbness. Amazed at her new feeling of comfort and control when she emerged from the trance state, she asked for some orange juice to drink and had no trouble retaining it. That evening she ate a light meal. The next day, after a good sleep, she was able to go home directly from the intensive-care unit.

"There is no doubt that without hypnosis," Spiegel says, "this woman would eventually have mobilized her resources and recovered," but, with her stress and desperate need for support, she used the trance experience to pull herself together quickly. "In this instance, the intervention with hypnosis made a long dialogue about this dilemma unnecessary."

A long dialogue, of course, is what Spiegel had been trained for. As a psychoanalyst, he could fully expect to spend weeks, months, and even years with a patient before being satisfied, if at all, with the treatment result. Unlike a surgeon, who may frequently achieve an on-the-spot cure, a psychoanalyst rarely has the satisfaction of seeing a patient come through the door with a serious problem and walk out healed soon afterward.

Spiegel had become well established as an analyst in the 1950s. He was not satisfied, however, that analysis was the best he could do for his patients. Lengthy therapy was often successful, but for some patients it was a waste of their money and his time. "I saw the impossibility," he recalls, "of making a major project out of every case that came along. I wasn't angry at analysis; I just wanted something more effective. The results I was getting with hypnosis were enviable compared to long-term therapy." He believed he could do more good for more people by more parsimonious means. "The truth, of course, is that I never was an orthodox analyst. At the White Institute, I found that I had an allergy to orthodoxy."

His views did not sit well with his fellow psychoanalysts. To some, he was "Herb the Heretic." For one thing, he discounted the notion that there is a single root to a problem that will explain all and solve all if only the patient and the analyst persevere in unearthing it. "There are many roots," he insists. "What we try to do is find *a* root that is relevant to the current issue and by resolving that we may get a ripple effect that helps other things too. If we do that, then that's as good as we can do. This idea that there is such a thing as being completely analyzed, thus totally freeing yourself of all anxieties, is just sheer nonsense."

Gradually, beginning in the 1950s, he cut down on analysis and devoted more of his time to patients who could benefit by short-term therapy. To a considerable extent, Spiegel became a kind of clinical court of last resort, seeing people with problems that persisted despite their own attempts to resolve them and despite the best efforts of the medical professionals who tried to help. Some individuals had been afflicted for the greater part of their lives, and yet, all the while, unknown to themselves, they possessed the means to master their difficulties. Eventually, because of the Hypnotic Induction Profile and imaginative treatment strategies, he was able to reduce drastically the number of therapy sessions for most patients. For some, a single session was sufficient if they demonstrated a capacity to heal themselves.

Spiegel was well ahead of his time. Today, many analysts have phased out exclusive use of analysis and have turned to less time-consuming therapies. Leading figures in the profession now recommend limited treatment and urge analysts to abandon their passive role and confront their patients more often.

Hypnosis, Spiegel had found, was particularly suitable for providing rapid resolution of conflicts that appear without warning for some violent reason. In this kind of emergency, he says, "situational stress enhances the proneness of a person to enter into the trance state."

One memorable case was that of a forty-year-old woman who was raped by a man who had entered her apartment while she slept. He had fled because of her screams and was not caught. The woman returned to work the following day and tried to regard the matter as "a nightmare that is all over," but she became increasingly distraught as the days passed. She had to be sent home from the office because of her outbursts of crying. When friends brought her to Spiegel a week after the rape, she was confused, tearful, and showing signs of panic.

Because of revealing pauses as the woman related the episode to him, he felt that she was trying to remember details that eluded her. Under hypnosis she was able to provide the missing information and did so with much emotion. It seems that even as she was resisting the rapist she was sexually aroused. In Spiegel's words, "She was reminded of her own need for physical and sexual closeness" after living alone for a year following a separation from her husband. Her description of the rape was a mixture of horror about the assault and fantasy about being loved.

During the week after the attack, Spiegel says, "she gradually realized that her temporary acceptance of this physical and sensuous excitement so offended her sense of moral decency that she berated herself for allowing this feeling to occur and feared she was degraded and perverted. This accounted for her delayed symptoms."

He was able to put things into perspective for her while she was still in trance and thus in a highly attentive and receptive frame of mind. Far from accepting her attacker, he pointed out, she had screamed; she had driven him away. There had merely been "an accidental uncovering of an understandable human feeling that had been dormant." Her fears that she was degraded were not founded upon fact but simply represented a confusion of issues.

After she was brought out of trance, they reviewed the events again. "She experienced a great sense of relief when she was able to tell me that her sexual excitement was understandable but in no way did it indicate that she desired such an experience in such a setting or that she condoned this man's intrusion. She lit up a cigarette, sighed several times, and jokingly referred to what an ordeal she had been through. Within another five or ten minutes she became composed and with a kind of gaiety remarked several times how unbelievable it was that she could feel so relieved within the course of an hour and a half. When she rejoined the two friends who had brought her, the expressions on their faces indicated their amazement at the drastic change that had occurred. She said to her friends, 'Let's go home and have a drink.' "

7

THE COLUMBIA COURSE

The art of medicine consists in three things:
the disease, the patient, and the physician.
The patient must combat the disease along
with the physician.

—HIPPOCRATES

One morning in 1964, in the hospital dining room at the Brookhaven Research Laboratories on Long Island, Dr. John E. Jesseph sat at a table drinking his fifth consecutive cup of coffee. "What am I doing?" he asked himself. "Why am I drinking so much coffee? I don't even like coffee."

Dr. Jesseph is now Professor of Surgery and Chairman of the Department of Surgery at the Indiana University School of Medicine. He remembers that occasion at Brookhaven as "a moment of truth" about his work that sparked his interest in hypnosis.

He was consuming so much coffee, Jesseph admitted to himself at the time, because he couldn't bear to get up and go to the ward where he did his research. There he would once again have to face the twenty-five women who were dying of metastatic breast cancer. They were participants in a program financed by the Atomic Energy Commission that was seeking to develop new radiation techniques for the treatment of cancer. Jesseph was feeling increasingly gloomy about his work with terminally ill patients because he could do little to lift their spirits and the only way he could ease their pain was to give them drugs that made them listless.

With such thoughts in mind, he came upon an announcement about a postgraduate course in clinical hypnosis being offered at Columbia University's College of Physicians and Surgeons. A psychiatrist, Herbert Spiegel, was the doctor in charge. Dr. Jesseph signed up for what he describes today as "an absolutely fascinating experience." For seven Saturdays in a row, he made the long journey into the city to immerse himself in a subject that had scarcely been mentioned in his years of medical training. (Spiegel's course was later split into basic and advanced sessions, each lasting a week, at different times in the year so that busy doctors from distant parts of the United States and abroad could attend. In 1982 Spiegel compressed his teachings into a single, intensive weeklong course given at the New York Academy of Medicine in upper Manhattan.)

Dr. Jesseph was so stimulated by what he learned that after the fifth Saturday session he began teaching cancer patients how to use their trance capacity to alter their perception of pain. Two weeks later, on the final day of the course, he had some interesting results to report. Though his patients varied, of course, in their hypnotic abilities, all of them had benefited to some extent by the relaxing-imagining suggestions he gave them and by self-hypnosis. As a group, they had reduced their use of painkilling drugs by two thirds. Their reports of nightmares had decreased by 90 percent. The heavy mood of the cancer ward had vanished. "And as for myself," Jesseph concluded, "I have gone back to drinking one cup of coffee in the morning."

Dr. Spiegel visited the hospital several months later. He

was impressed by the sight of patients reading, knitting, and playing bridge with each other while maintaining their individual trance states. He remembers it today as "a strangely serene atmosphere."

Until recent times, it was difficult for a doctor like John Jesseph to acquire professional training in hypnosis. When Spiegel began private practice after World War II, hypnosis was mostly in the hands of people outside organized medicine. "I remember going to meetings of hypnotists in those days," he says, "and coming away feeling very disturbed. So many of them were really weird characters who had come out of the woodwork. They seemed to think that they belonged to some kind of secret society and that they were the privileged possessors of a mysterious force that they could impose on other people. I just felt so uncomfortable. I felt that, dammit, if hypnosis has value, it should be done out in the daylight by medical professionals."

What was needed was a regular course on hypnosis given at a leading medical school by a physician with impeccable credentials. Spiegel was given the chance to start such a course at the College of Physicians and Surgeons in 1961. It has been going ever since and it has set the standard for the instruction in medical hypnosis that is available today at Harvard, Stanford, the Walter Reed Army Medical Center, and other pacesetting institutions around the country.

"The reason I'm at Columbia today," Spiegel relates, "is that back in 1960 the Orthopedic Department at Columbia Presbyterian Hospital was at a loss about what to do with a woman whose leg had been paralyzed for a year and a half. After trying a number of things that didn't work they called in a psychiatrist, Bill Horwitz, for his opinion. He suspected that the paralysis was hysterical. For one thing, when he used Pentothol the stiffness disappeared for a while but it returned when the effects of the drug wore off.

"As it turned out, he was exactly right. We didn't know it at the time, but she got this paralysis because of watching her beautiful son, who was nine or ten years old, fade away and die over an eleven-month period. He had a congenital defect in his pancreas. At his funeral she overheard someone criticizing her because she wasn't crying. In fact, she had cried herself out during the previous year. Three months later, because she was still apathetic about the whole thing, some neighbors gave her a party to cheer her up. She slipped on the patio and when she got up her back was bent. It was diagnosed as a disk problem. They took a disk out even though it wasn't necessary. The back problem was just a somatic metaphor. It symbolized her troubles and worries. While she was recovering in the hospital they put one leg in traction. Later, when they took the apparatus off, the leg was stiff and paralyzed and it stayed that way.

"Horwitz had the idea that hypnosis might work in this case but he knew that the neurologists and the psychoanalysts at Columbia Presbyterian would object. They wouldn't want to get tainted with anything so bizarre as hypnosis. Fortunately, Frank Stinchfield, the head of the Orthopedic Department at the time, was a very secure professional. When Horwitz said, 'I think this is hysteria and I know a guy in the city who can do hypnosis,' Stinchfield told him, 'Hell, yes, if you think it can work, let's try it.' So I was brought in on the case.

"I found the woman to be highly hypnotizable. In my first session with her, she was able to develop a tremor in the paralyzed leg. That leg was tremendously swollen because she hadn't used it for a year and a half. The muscles had atrophied. I gave her a posthypnotic signal that she would be able to bring on a movement in the leg. We went on in this way for weeks. The swelling went down as the movements increased. Eventually there was full recovery."

The case became the talk of the hospital. For Columbia Presbyterian, it was the beginning of acceptance of hypnosis as a legitimate treatment modality. The more secure and self-confident the institution, Spiegel has found, the more likely it will try something different. He began to get more calls from doctors who had baffling cases and were stumped about what to do next. After a while, he was invited to lecture on hypnosis to the resident physicians at Columbia Presbyterian. Then he was asked to give talks at staff meetings.

"It was always done informally, however," he says. "After nearly two years of this I said that if hypnosis is valuable enough for the hospital to use and for me to teach, then I want an appointment." He was invited to join the faculty and conduct an annual course on hypnosis. His first students were Columbia's own residents and interns, but outside physicians were admitted the following year. Today, two decades later, enrollment for the course is higher than ever as medical hypnosis comes into its own.

Among the first practitioners to sign up for the course was Dr. Ernest E. Rockey, now associate clinical professor of surgery at New York Medical College. At the time he was already well established in his field. In fact, as a surgeon with a special interest in the chest and lungs, he was recognized as a pioneer for having developed a method for draining the lungs of patients with extreme forms of emphysema. He had devised an ingenious surgical procedure that opened a channel in the trachea or windpipe, making it possible for the patient himself, by inserting a tube through the tiny window in his throat, to extract excess phlegm. The patient could do it at home periodically instead of going to the hospital for a complicated draining ritual.

The nature of the illness, however, meant that the tracheal fenestration operation was hazardous to the patient under general anesthesia. It usually was done with a local that did not completely block the pain. The discomfort was great and the operation was strenuous for both patient and surgeon.

"Because of the appalling ignorance about hypnosis within the medical profession," Dr. Rockey says, "it took me until 1962 to discover that there was such a thing as medical hypnosis and to find Dr. Spiegel." It so happened that Rockey had a tracheal fenestration operation scheduled while he was attending the Columbia course. His patient was an old friend who was willing to take a chance with hypnosis as the sole anesthetic agent. Rockey was delighted to find that he could cut into the throat tissues without hurting the patient. It was his easiest operation ever. When the time came to bring his friend out of the trance, he first assured him that he would feel very comfortable and experience no pain during the recovery period. Moreover, he would be able to eat right away because of the ease of swallowing. Most patients could not eat for the first three days after the operation because of the pain of swallowing.

"When he opened his eyes," Rockey remembers, "the first thing he said was, 'I'm hungry.' He proceeded to eat a hearty lunch. This had never happened before with any patient. It was the most impressive experience we ever had."

It was also a turning point in Dr. Rockey's career. Viewing hypnosis as "a godsend for the respiratory patient," he began to employ it in his throat operations whenever a patient proved to be sufficiently hypnotizable. With experience, he learned that he did not have to go to great lengths to make sure that the patient's trance would hold during surgery. "In the early days," he says, "I would hypnotize the patient well in advance of surgery, personally escort him to the operating room, and insist that everyone else be absolutely silent while I maintained a steady stream of chatter to reassure the patient—and myself—that all was well. None of this was necessary. Once the patient is in trance and you've told him to pay attention only to yourself, he doesn't listen to anyone else. It doesn't matter if there are observers in the room talking about the operation—and I get a lot of them who still can't believe what they're seeing. There was one old-time nurse who slipped into the operating room without saying anything and lifted up the drapes around the operating table to see if we had some secret device to give Pentothol to the patient. Then she walked out, saying, 'I still don't believe it.' "

Dr. Rockey became an enthusiast for medical hypnosis and a regular lecturer at the Columbia course. In his personal life, as an average hypnotic subject, he has made good use of self-hypnosis, particularly when visiting his dentist. "I can ask him to do everything at one sitting and then settle back in the chair for an hour or two of rest." On one occasion, he relied on his trance capacity to counter the pain during a seventy-five-minute abscessed-tooth operation. "Everything was fine until the surgeon told me that he was about to cut out a piece of bone. I got scared. But then I imagined that Dr. Spiegel was hypnotizing me. I could see him even though he wasn't there. It went marvelously."

Although convinced that every physician "will one day learn the art of trance," Rockey does not present hypnosis to his fellow surgeons as a replacement for standard forms of anesthesia in the operating room. "We have wonderful anesthesiologists in our hospitals," he says, "and in most cases there is no need for hypnoanesthesia unless the patient requests it and has enough trance capacity. But if an operation is risky with chemical anesthesia, then that's a different story." Spiegel's view on this subject is that "every good anesthesia department works on the principle that you have a variety of ways to do the job. Hypnosis can be seen as one of the alternatives. As with any procedure, if it's not working you shift to something else. Every time we use hypnosis for an operation, an anesthesiologist is present to do the monitoring so he's around to try something else if need be."

The value of hypnosis in reducing preoperative anxieties and enhancing postoperative recovery should be obvious, Rockey says, but he also describes it as supremely useful for what he calls "preventive surgery." Because he believes that most of his lung-disease operations would not have been necessary if the patients had known how to protect their bodies in the first place, he sets aside a number of hours each week for the teaching of self-hypnosis to patients who wish to quit smoking. One young woman told him she wanted to give up cigarettes but not marijuana. "I enjoy it too much," she explained. Rockey proposed that she put herself into a trance and see if she could use her imagination to re-create the sensations she had felt during her most recent experience with marijuana. "It worked!" she exclaimed afterward. "I got the effect of grass without smoking any!"

Dr. Rockey's preventive surgery is a reflection of the emphasis that is placed on preventive medicine at the hypnosis course. During one recent session, Spiegel told the doctors: "If I had a chance to give a perspective while we're spending a week talking about therapy, I'd like to have the word 'prevention' written all the way across the stage and the word 'therapy' way down there on the bottom so you could barely see it. As physicians in our community, we need a sense of perspective so that we don't get so lost in what we're doing that we fail to see that it is trivial compared to the bigger issues of society. Simple things like people eating more sensibly, getting exercise, and not smoking would probably eliminate 50 percent of the private practice of doctors in this country. People would be so much healthier. Yet medical schools don't stress that. Those doctors who are interested in preventive medicine have a hard time getting access to students. It's very difficult to get research grants for this because the establishment is much more concerned about medical gimmickry."

Spiegel, who is not one to pull his punches, tells the physicians that "some of the dumbest people in the world are doctors, and certainly some of the most antipsychological people in the world are doctors. They are so influenced by hard science that they think and act like plumbers, electricians, and carpenters. They discount anything they can't measure or see under a microscope. They'll turn to a pill or a knife or a gadget before even considering that the patient's mind might be more helpful than anything. An anesthesiologist at a medical school once told me that 'the human body is a chemical box and our job is understanding the chemical equilibrium and seeing that things are in balance.' There was no recognition at all of psychological factors."

In a Chicago hospital, he recalls, a patient who was dying of cancer of the cervix was in terrible pain. "The resident there had just learned to do the Profile and he was delighted to find that she was a Four. He showed her how to develop numbness for her pain. For the first time in months she had no pain. There was just this numb feeling. She was able to get up and walk about. One of the nurses actually cried when she saw this woman walking down the corridor. When the resident in neurosurgery came in on a Monday and saw her walking around, he questioned whether they should still go ahead with the spinal cord operation scheduled for Wednesday. He called the chief surgeon, a real prima donna, who was furious. He wanted to know who was interfering with his schedule. 'She's due for surgery Wednesday,' he said, 'and, dammit, she's going to get it.' When he came in and saw the patient, he told her, 'Young lady, don't fool yourself. You've got real pain and you need this surgery.' She immediately collapsed and felt the pain all over again."

When Spiegel began his Columbia course, the belief that there was something weak-minded about being hypnotizable was so deep-seated that he carefully avoided using the attending doctors as hypnotic subjects. He relied on cooperative patients and other nonprofessionals to demonstrate trance. "The doctors would have been insulted," he says, "if you told them that they could be hypnotized. And they'd be terribly embarrassed if they went into trance in front of their colleagues. Now the picture is entirely different. They complain if we neglect to measure their trance capacity."

These days, all of the two hundred doctors who come to upper Manhattan for basic training in clinical hypnosis sit down with Spiegel or one of his associates early in the week to see where they rank on the scale of hypnotizability. There is no lack of volunteers for the onstage demonstrations of trance. During a coffee break or the lunch hour, when a buffet of sandwiches and salads is provided, a dozen or more doctors may be seen comparing eye rolls or hypnotizing each other just for practice. The Profile scores of the physicians reveal that they have about the same proportion of zero-to-five hypnotic personalities as the general public. During the demonstrations of trance induction the most trance-prone of the physicians in the audience occasionally reveal themselves by the way their arms automatically rise in unison with the arm levitation of the subject being hypnotized. Spiegel advises highly hypnotizable clinicians to recognize their own inclination to spontaneous trance states and to keep out of hypnosis themselves when they lead their patients into trance. "After all," he tells them, "somebody's got to be in charge. You don't want to be like an anesthesiologist who whiffs the same ether he gives his patient."

It is not uncommon for a doctor at the course to observe Spiegel demonstrating a trance strategy with a patient and take that strategy more to heart than he or she realizes. On one occasion, a psychiatrist paid particular attention to Spiegel's stop-smoking technique because she was herself a heavy smoker. She listened closely as the subject in trance was told that his innocent body deserves respect and needs to be protected from poisonous smoke. A few hours later, while driving home from the course, the psychiatrist was astonished and momentarily frightened when her hand went into spasms as she reached into her pocketbook for her cigarettes. After first thinking that something was physically wrong with her, she realized that her hand was giving her a message. The shaking started whenever she reached for the cigarettes and stopped as soon as she withdrew her hand. She became a nonsmoker on the spot.

Another doctor told this story at the advanced course in medical hypnosis: "When I took the basic course a few months ago, I was a smoker but I had no particular urge to give it up because I actually only smoked at work. It only amounted to a few cigarettes a day. I didn't think it was much of a problem. After the course, whenever I picked up a cigarette I found that I only smoked half of it. Then two weeks after that, whenever I picked up a cigarette I couldn't smoke it at all. I really haven't given up smoking but my body has. I would like to go on smoking but my body doesn't want to."

David Spiegel, who led the discussion about this experience, observed that "this is an example of how the message gets across on a whole variety of levels. Cognitive understanding is just one level. The doctor actually paid more attention to the suggestion about smoking as poison than he realized. He absorbed the message without really thinking about it. His body knew what was good for him even if he didn't."

Herbert Spiegel encourages the doctors to share such experiences because he wants them to think of hypnosis not just in terms of the formal encounter of hypnotist and subject but as a phenomenon that happens to people more than they know and as a human resource that is eminently useful and always available. During one recent session of the course, a physician stood up to say: "I tried to eat a sandwich yesterday and I felt a terrible twinge in a tooth that had been bothering me for quite a while. Fortunately, my husband is a dentist so I asked him to grind the tooth. This is something I usually find very painful. I had never used hypnosis before but I thought I'd give it a try. I relied on my memory and tried to re-create the feeling I once had when I had a badly cramped toe. I concentrated on that feeling so much that I couldn't feel the actual work being done on the tooth. I was aware of the passage of time and what was going on but there was no pain. Later on, when my husband asked me about the tooth, I could only say that it felt as if it were saying, 'I'm trying to hurt.' "

Another doctor went to the stage to tell what happened when he was tested for his trance capacity. He said he had been reluctant to be hypnotized because of the arm-levitation feature of the test. Four years earlier, he explained, he had seriously injured his left arm in a skiing accident. Ever since, he had felt a good deal of pain when he raised it too high. "I went ahead with the hypnosis anyway," he said, "and it was the left arm that floated. When the trance was over I was told that the arm had gone all the way up in the air. That was really strange to me because that was something I had not been able to do in four years."

Such personal accounts help give the course its spontaneous and unpredictable quality even though Spiegel and his ensemble of teaching assistants and lecturers work to a finely tuned schedule. He is seen as something of a high-wire artist by the doctors because he demonstrates hypnosis with volunteers he has never seen before and he presents as live case histories patients he has not rehearsed. Usually he has no idea how they will describe their experiences with hypnosis or respond to audience questions. Said one man as he looked about the auditorium, "I thought you asked me here because I haven't paid my bill."

Spiegel remains unruffled when he is unable to hypnotize a volunteer; it gives him the chance to make the point that some people simply cannot go into trance. And if a former patient confesses, for example, that she controlled her weight with self-hypnosis for many months but no longer, it is his opportunity to talk about the importance of motivation and to say the obvious: that there are no guarantees of short-term or long-term success with this or any other medical procedure. Furthermore, there are some things, like extreme alcoholism and drug addiction, that generally are impervious to a hypnotic approach because patients have such difficulty maintaining concentration. A highly hypnotizable person, however, who is caught up in a destructive environment because he was easily influenced might well be helped to get out of it by hypnotic countersuggestions and changes in his way of life.

"Don't think of yourself as a failure if hypnosis doesn't work," Spiegel tells the doctors. "Just go on and try something else. In some situations, especially with habit control, it is really up to the patient once you've shown him what he can do for himself. There are times when my view is, 'If you don't care, I don't care, and when you do care, let me know.' I'm not going to be embarrassed if I show someone how to stop smoking and he starts smoking again. I'd only be embarrassed if I didn't know how to show him what to do."

Knowledge of hypnosis in terms of the varying capacities of people can sometimes give a doctor the means to help a patient deal with a supposed defeat. David Spiegel learned from an obstetrician about a woman who was emotionally upset because she had asked for chemical anesthesia when giving birth. "She and her husband had faithfully attended courses in the Lamaze techniques for painless childbirth. Now she felt like a failure because she couldn't tolerate the pain. If other women could do it, what was wrong with her? We found out that she was low in hypnotic capacity. The Lamaze ritual has a lot in common with hypnosis so she could hardly be expected to respond as well as women with a lot of trance talent. She was no failure; she was just being herself."

It is not uncommon for a practitioner to travel across the country to learn about hypnosis from Spiegel and discover that he has been employing a form of hypnosis all along. A clinical psychologist from Minneapolis, for example, told of using "a dissociation technique" in his practice: "When I find myself getting caught in a very cognitive conversation with a patient, and I'm trying to get in touch with his feelings, I will routinely close my eyes, roll them up, and take fifteen or twenty seconds to just go inside myself in an empathetic mode and try to imagine where to contact that person simply in terms of feelings. I see now that I switch to a Dionysian mode of functioning in a very explicit way."

Dr. Bernard Stern, a Manhattan internist who says that "the course transformed all my work," testifies that "the real eye-opener was the realization that I had been using hypnosis during all of my quarter century in medicine without knowing it. Not as formal trance inductions but in the real sense of getting in touch with patients. I started in practice when I was twenty-five but I looked even younger. New patients would ask me, 'Where's your father?' So I made it my business to be especially careful in talking to patients and explaining things to them so that I could get through and motivate them, especially if they were facing something like major surgery. If a patient is calm and is really concentrating on what you're saying, and if you have put him in a positive frame of mind, that, to me, is hypnosis without formal trance and I had been doing it all along.

"Among other things, the course has given me a way of dealing with patients who have crazy ideas about hypnosis. They've seen it on the stage and they are afraid of going under and being made to look foolish. But if you ask them if they would like to learn a method of concentrating and relaxing, that's different. When talking about their capacity for hypnosis, I tell them that it's like checking out your musical ability: 'Maybe you have it; maybe you don't; maybe you're a musical genius.' I make sure there's no contest between us. 'If you don't want to be hypnotized, then it's not going to happen.' I get rid of the notion that this is something I do to the patient. Hypnosis is something he can do for himself.

"As it happens, almost all my patients want to try hypnosis, and that's great because I find I can do more for them now, sometimes with very dramatic results, without having to advise medication. I used to feel so frustrated whenever I had to turn to pills. One of my patients was an elderly woman who had developed an intestinal obstruction. The X rays revealed that one of her vertebrae was completely collapsed and pressing on her spinal cord. The nerves that came out of that area went to the intestinal tract among other places. She was in terrible pain and there was still a lot of pain after the operation, so she was getting a lot of narcotics. In fact, she was becoming addicted. Her eye roll was only a one, very low, but I knew she was health-food conscious and was interested in things like hypnosis, so I asked her if she'd like to give it a try. She was able to go into trance and I gave her a strategy for relieving the pain.

"When I saw her a week later, she said she had not taken a single narcotic tablet all week long, just an occasional aspirin. We did hypnosis again for reinforcement. A week later, she came to the office. I was prepared for a relapse but she said she had quit the aspirins as well as the narcotics. She had fired her nurse. She was walking a lot and becoming more active. Weeks later, she was still going strong. I asked her for some details about her self-hypnosis. I had suggested that she get a feeling of numbness for the pain by going into trance and imagining icebergs up in the Arctic. She was still doing that but she had added something of her own. She said she puts her hands on her abdomen and feels the heat from her hands going right through her abdomen into the nerves and the pain just goes. I said to her, 'In other words, you make a heating pad out of your hands.' She said, 'That's right, and it works!' "

Dr. Frederick Dick, an internist at Columbia Presbyterian Medical Center, is another physician whose work was transformed by hypnotic knowledge. Many years ago, as a smoker who consumed three to four packs of cigarettes a day, he sought out Spiegel to see if hypnosis could help him with his habit. "To my absolute surprise," he says, "I never picked up another cigarette after one forty-five-minute session. That inspired me to take the course.

"The big discovery for me in medicine the longer I practice is how much the mind is in control, and how I have come to write fewer and fewer prescriptions. In the last ten years I have reduced to one-tenth the number of prescriptions for sleeping medications. As for tranquilizers, I point out to the patient that the most magnificent tranquilizer he can use is this ability to relax and float."

Dr. Harold Wain, a regular lecturer at the course, describes the uses of hypnosis at his pain clinic at Walter Reed Army Medical Center. "Every patient who comes to the clinic gets the Profile," he says, "and every patient who gets evaluated on our liaison service is asked to do an eye roll that is recorded on a chart. Every psychiatric resident at Walter Reed gets a twenty-four-hour course on hypnosis that is based on the Spiegel course.

"We find out the trance abilities and personalities of our pain patients and create appropriate strategies. We once had a two-star general who had residual surgical pain. He was low in trance ability, so we gave him a cognitive strategy. Since he was in the habit of giving orders, we told him to *order* the pain away. The pain obeyed.

"Then there was the nurse who was very athletic. She played a lot of softball and always took a shower after a game. She was also very hypnotizable. We taught her how to head off her migraine headaches by taking a cold hypnotic shower every two hours. All she had to do was take a few seconds to go into trance and imagine a cooling numbness from the cold water pouring down on her.

"Another patient was a thirteen-year-old boy who had been having terrible migraine headaches for five years. Because he liked to travel in airplanes, the strategy with him was to have him go into self-hypnosis and imagine being a passenger on a plane and directing a stream of cold air on his head from the air conditioner. It worked beautifully, especially after he added to the strategy himself by going into the imaginary plane, taking down the No Smoking Zone signs, and replacing them with his own No Headache Zone signs."

By no means does every clinician who takes the course go on to use hypnosis as a major part of his or her practice. Some may simply use their newfound knowledge of the eye roll and of variations in hypnotic capacity to better understand the personalities of their patients. In the case of Dr. John Jesseph, who had such success with his cancer patients at Brookhaven, he finds in his work as a surgeon that only occasionally does he do a trance induction ("It's great if you very quickly want to get an arm on a problem or if what you need is an honest-to-God change of behavior") yet he frequently resorts to simple suggestion or relaxation techniques. "I'm a surgeon, not a psychiatrist," he says, "but at least I know in dealing with patients with terrible anxieties that there are some very effective parahypnotic ways of calming them down and reassuring them."

No matter what use they make of hypnosis after taking the course, it is a great leap forward, Spiegel feels, if the doctors now look at their patients in a new light: as people whose feelings count and whose resources for self-healing are greater than had been imagined. By his every word and action, Spiegel conveys a message of the value of a doctor-patient partnership in healing—with the patient more than just a junior partner. On one occasion, while describing a young woman's success in mobilizing her trance capacity to rid herself of a loathsome skin disease, he commented that "this patient reminds us that we are not as important or as necessary as we like to think we are. The goal of good therapy is to make the doctor unnecessary as quickly as possible."

He agrees with Dr. Michael Crichton, the Harvard-trained physician and author (*The Andromeda Strain, The Terminal Man*), that the scientific orientation of American medical education "takes incoming medical students who are interested in people and transforms them into doctors interested in disease." Said Crichton in a *New York Times* Op-Ed page article: the practicing doctor with his years of training behind him "makes two disquieting discoveries. First, he finds that he must practice a great deal of unscientific medicine—dealing with the 70 percent of his patients who have no demonstrable illness, but varying complaints. This calls for behavioral training which he almost certainly lacks. Second, he discovers that his training is rapidly outdated but the refresher courses run by university doctors are generally abstruse, heavily scientific, and lacking the practical details on patient care that he needs."

The paradox of the Columbia course is that it is about as practical and people-oriented as postgraduate medical instruction can be while at the same time, as an exercise in teaching hypnosis, it is unique in its concern for method, discipline, and scientific rigor. Unusual attention is paid to the identification of hypnotizable and nonhypnotizable individuals, to the assessment of their trance capacities and psychological intactness, and to the selection of treatment strategies to match the differing trance styles of patients. "In an organized, systematic way," Spiegel says, "using the Hypnotic Induction Profile, we are putting into operation what many experienced therapists do with the seat of their pants. A really good doctor sizes up his patients and knows that a treatment that will work for one person may not work for someone else even if he has the identical problem."

It is ironic, Spiegel continues, that "this not very reputable thing called hypnosis, which people think of as mysterious and unscientific, can now be used as an instrument for a practitioner to make a rational, logical, diagnostic decision about whether a patient will be responsive to any kind of therapy, and if so, which kind."

He takes a dim view of "these cults that have come into the field of therapy and therapists who lock themselves into a single technique for all patients and all complaints." He tells the doctors that "our thesis is that there is no kind of therapy, even witchcraft, that isn't useful to somebody somehow somewhere some way on some occasion. It's just dumb luck if a doctor who's got one way to deal with all problems comes up with a certain number of successes. The real professional tries to make a reasonable diagnosis as to which kind of therapy is best for the individual. One of my patients a few years ago was a very simple, very superstitious woman who came to me with insomnia. She was convinced that her sister in Haiti was sticking pins in a doll and that's why she couldn't sleep. I referred her to a witch doctor I knew about in the Bronx. He, very appropriately, wouldn't see her right away. She had to come to him on a certain night when the moon was a certain way, and she had to appear in a white gown and so on. She went through a ritual with several other people. By morning it was all over and she slept. There was no more insomnia. I was proud of that referral. I felt I was doing good medicine."

As a teacher of medical hypnosis, Dr. Spiegel is anything but dogmatic. He cheerfully describes his own experience with trance in therapy, demonstrates the methods he has found effective, offers the Hypnotic Induction Profile as a means for measuring and monitoring trance capacity—and then encourages the doctors to go ahead and use hypnosis in any way that works best for their patients and themselves. He even makes a point of exposing them to experts in the field whose opinions and techniques contradict his own.

"Our guidelines are not meant to be dictatorial," he says. "Rules can be broken. I have enormous respect for the many doctors around the world who have good therapeutic sense and use hypnosis with an intuitive, free-wheeling style that can often be very, very effective. They may not be able to explain how they get their results; we may only hear about their successes; but we can still appreciate the sharpness of their clinical skills."

For a number of years, until it became too difficult for him to travel to New York from his home in Arizona, the late Dr. Milton Erickson—once described in the press as "the foxy grandpa of American hypnotism"—was a guest lecturer at the Columbia course. Spiegel admired Erickson for his pioneering work in medical hypnosis and for the way he coped with a host of infirmities—everything from dyslexia and arrhythmia to color blindness and tone deafness. He was twice stricken with polio, in his teens and in middle age. He was described as the archetype of the wounded physician who helps others by struggling to heal himself. The trance state became Erickson's refuge from the pain that so constantly assailed him. "I just go into trance," he once explained, "saying, 'Unconscious, do your stuff!' "

Spiegel and Erickson agreed on some aspects of hypnosis. Erickson's view that it is "a state of intensified attention and receptiveness, and an increased responsiveness to an idea or to a set of ideas" was in accord with Spiegel's definition. Both men emphasized that far too much attention has been placed on the actions of the hypnotist to secure trances and too little on what the subject is doing and experiencing. "The development of a trance state," Erickson said in his book *Advanced Techniques of Hypnosis and Therapy*, "is an intrapsychic phenomenon dependent on internal processes, and the activity of the hypnotist serves only to create a favorable situation. As an analogy, an incubator supplies a favorable environment for the hatching of eggs but the actual hatching derives from the development of life processes within the egg."

They both agreed that most people use only a fraction of their mental abilities. When faced with problems, said Erickson, people rely on their conscious attitudes—the things they have been taught, the things they "know"—without realizing that "there is a greater wealth of stored material in the unconscious" and that "their unconscious is smarter than they are."

Spiegel differed with Erickson, however, about the way to get patients to bypass the conscious mind and reach the storehouse of the unconscious. In contrast to Spiegel's elementary and almost matter-of-fact approach when doing a trance induction, as if applying the architectural principle of "less is more," Erickson over the course of half a century developed a bewildering variety of ploys, tricks, and verbal and nonverbal techniques for bringing on the trance state. In his use of hypnosis, he turned to such things as shock, surprise, paradox, double binds, and shifting frames of reference. He was known to hypnotize a patient by ignoring him completely as he carried on a conversation with another person—a conversation loaded with trance suggestions that the patient picked up.

By insisting that he could hypnotize anyone, Erickson took issue with Spiegel's contention that a significant number of people, for biological or psychological reasons, are barely hypnotizable or cannot go into trance at all. As they jousted with each other before the doctors, Spiegel would venture that a number of these people might succumb to Erickson's tactics and shift into hypnosis but that others, out of sheer exasperation or exhaustion, might simply simulate the trance state. He once challenged Erickson to induce hypnosis with a patient who had profiled as a Zero. After half an hour, Spiegel called off the exercise because the patient still was not hypnotized and the doctors in the audience were obviously bored.

"We used to battle with each other in this way," Spiegel recalls, "but it was always friendly combat. I wanted the doctors to have the experience of seeing a legendary charismatic therapist at work, just doing hypnosis without measuring ability or recording how well performance matches potential." In recent years, a dynamic general practitioner from Hellertown, Pennsylvania, Dr. L. S. Wolfe, better known as Pete Wolfe, has made regular appearances at the course so that Spiegel can present "an example of the superb seat-of-the-pants clinician whose whole approach is the antithesis of what we teach here."

Now in his early sixties, Dr. Wolfe is a creative and unorthodox physician with a distinctive clinical style. He is not a hypnotherapist; he is a therapist who uses hypnosis when he feels it is warranted. On occasion, he employs acupuncture, a procedure that he says has little if anything to do with precise needle placement and everything to do with hypnosis.

"Some of my patients," he says, "come to me simply because they have heard that I am a GP who does hypnosis. They arrive with their own beliefs about it. They equate trance with cure. So much so that sometimes I don't even have to make any therapeutic suggestions. A patient with eczema, for example, goes into trance and when I see him a week later the eczema is gone. He is grateful to me but I didn't have anything to do with it. I might con my patients sometimes but I don't con myself."

Wolfe agrees with Spiegel that there is a range of hypnotizability, but he ignores it. "I used to worry when I came across a patient who was impervious to hypnosis but now I don't pay attention to it. I just go right ahead. As far as I'm concerned, it's this bullying self-confidence I have that makes everybody hypnotizable."

Whether or not all of Dr. Wolfe's hypnotized patients are actually in a formal trance state, Spiegel comments, "the seemingly miraculous cures he often achieves are the result of many things: his stature, his commanding presence, his self-assurance, his reputation in the community, and even the sense of mystery that many people feel about hypnosis. In his gruff but tender way, he takes full advantage of the aura and the air of expectancy that the idea of hypnosis evokes."

Wolfe has the look of a marine drill sergeant. He stands—or towers—six feet, five inches. His face is rugged, his hair is closely cropped, and his manner is rough and ready. He speaks no medical jargon. He sometimes gets results—the kind of instant cures that are possible with psychosomatic illnesses—simply by telling a patient, "Do it!" Such a command, of course, can amount to an immediate trance induction as well as trance therapy for a well-motivated and hypnotically responsive person.

One of Dr. Wolfe's patients was a woman in such pain that he couldn't move her into the trance state—not until he suddenly embraced her and declared, "I love you!"

Her surprise was so great, it appears, that the pain momentarily diminished and he was able to hypnotize her and begin therapy. With children, he often does fast inductions simply by getting them settled and telling them, in a friendly but forceful manner, "Relax your bellybutton!" As the children focus on their bellybuttons, their bodies relax and they shift into trance.

In relating certain case histories, Wolfe sometimes wonders, along with his audience, whether what happened was hypnosis. "A woman came to me and told me that her children wanted a cat for Christmas but she couldn't give them a cat because one kid breaks out in hives and the other gets asthma. I told her to make a flat statement to the kids: 'If you want a cat for Christmas you can have it but there will be no hives and there will be no asthma.' She did this and they got the cat for Christmas. Three days later, the kids had hives and asthma. Again, following my instructions, she made a flat statement, 'Okay, that's it! The cat has to go!' This time the kids really got the message. The cat is still there but the hives and the asthma have gone. To me, that's hypnosis. Or else it's related to hypnosis. One thing for sure, I wouldn't have thought of doing that unless I had learned hypnosis. I found out about the power of suggestion and the control people have over their bodies."

Wolfe exhorts the doctors to use it on themselves. "A couple of years ago, I had to go to the hospital for an operation. The surgeon said I would have to stay in the hospital for a week after the operation and then I would have to stay home for a week. I asked him why. Because of the pain, he said. Is that the only reason? Yes, he said. Well, to me, the pain would be unrewarding pain; I wouldn't get any benefit out of it. I told the surgeon: With your permission, I'll go to work the day after surgery. Which I did. And I had no pain."

Dr. Wolfe runs a busy clinic. Many of his patients are on welfare or scrape along at low-income jobs. They are grateful to find an experienced physician who will, for a token fee, teach them in a few minutes how to take control of an ailment or affliction that may have plagued them for years and drained their resources. Having turned to general practice after a career as an anesthesiologist, Wolfe half-jokingly says that "I took up hypnosis because the cost in equipment is so low," but, in truth, he took it up because nothing else was so effective.

"Hypnosis is cheap," he tells the doctors. "It's quick and it works. If people are motivated, you'll be amazed at how well it works. And if it doesn't work, so what? There's everything to gain and nothing to lose."

It is this facet of hypnosis—an option worth trying that might well succeed, and no harm done if it doesn't—that gives Spiegel's course its optimistic atmosphere. Even the most cynical practitioner, as he observes patients using hypnotic self-control and hears other doctors speak of their experiences, cannot help but get the message that this is for real and that this is something that might make him a far more effective clinician than he had thought possible.

Dr. Wolfe warns the doctors to be ready for those occasions when hypnotic intervention brings about a sudden day-and-night change: "It's hair-raising when it happens to you the first few times." According to Dr. Jeffrey S. Tarte, an expert on the uses of hypnosis in dentistry, the great satisfaction about understanding trance is being able to turn to it when nothing else seems to work. He tells of the night he was called to the Eye and Ear Hospital in Manhattan to see if he could help a woman whose mouth wouldn't open. "We figured out afterward that it was a case of acute muscle spasm. The doctors had tried intravenous Valium and everything else short of prying her mouth open. When I found out that she was hypnotizable, I got her into a trance and told her she was getting so tired that she just had to sleep. Pretty soon she started to yawn. Her mouth opened as wide as it had ever been."

It was the sheer effectiveness of hypnosis as a medical tool that brought David Spiegel into the same field as his father despite an understandable early reluctance to toil in the same medical vineyard.

"I was still in my third year of medical school at Harvard," he remembers, "and working at Children's Hospital in Boston. There was a young woman who had been admitted for emergency treatment for the third time in as many months because of an unrelenting succession of asthma attacks. I could hear her wheezing all the way down the hall. She was hunched forward in bed, her knuckles white, her mother standing nearby wringing her hands. No one seemed to know what to do with her and neither did I until I thought of asking her if she would like to learn an exercise to help her with her breathing. When she agreed, I just asked her to close her eyes and let her body float and let one hand float up in the air, which it did. I said that each breath you take will be a little deeper and easier. This was the first time I had ever tried this procedure with a patient, and I wasn't too confident. To my amazement, and her mother's amazement, she began to relax. Within five minutes she was lying in the bed and breathing more easily all the time. The emergency was over. She was able to sleep.

"I was feeling pretty good about the whole thing until the resident and some of the other doctors took me to task for using something as unorthodox as hypnosis. They even wondered whether I had done something illegal, which wasn't true. Fortunately, both the patient and her mother were on my side so I was allowed to go ahead and teach her a simple self-hypnosis exercise so that she could ward off any future asthma attacks. All she had to do each time was shift into trance and imagine herself breathing cool mountain air. And it worked. I kept in touch with her for many years and she came to the course a few times to appear before the doctors. She not only mastered her asthma, using self-hypnosis regularly and medication occasionally, but she began a career as a respiratory therapist."

8

THE EYE ROLL

I perceived unequivocal signs of the mesmeric
influence. The glassy roll of the eye was
changed for that expression of uneasy *inward*
examination which is never seen except in
cases of sleep-walking.
—EDGAR ALLAN POE, "The Facts
in the Case of M. Valdemar"

At a symposium, "Obedience to Authority," held in a
ballroom of New York's Waldorf-Astoria Hotel one October morning in 1977, Herbert Spiegel listened carefully as
a fellow member of the panel of experts, former White
House counsel John Dean, described his role in the Watergate scandal.

The assembled psychiatrists, psychologists, and other
human behavior specialists were exploring a major twen-
tieth-century concern: the readiness of all too many people to follow orders even if they lead to illegal or
unethical acts.

As Spiegel heard Dean, a self-described "case study,"
speak unemotionally and analytically about first going
along with the Watergate cover-up and later breaking
away from the conspiracy for reasons of personal survival,
he felt that he was getting a good picture of the man's
personality. Dean sounded like an Apollonian; that is, a
person low on the scale of hypnotizability who could not
easily be fooled and who would always be reluctant to

surrender critical judgment. Spiegel was confident that Dean had a low eye roll.

Dean was equally intrigued by Spiegel and by what the psychiatrist had said in his address earlier that morning. Spiegel had approached the issue of obedience to authority by speaking of the special vulnerability of those people who appear to have a natural propensity for relinquishing their normal critical judgment and allowing themselves to be swayed by others. He called them Fours and Fives: highly hypnotizable personalities who could be identified by their ability to roll their eyes back into their heads. Unless a mental disturbance interfered with their capacity to maintain concentration, they were able to use formal hypnosis and self-hypnosis with unrivaled facility. That could be a great blessing. The negative side of their exceptional hypnotic talent, however, was a proneness to accept the reasoning and the directions of other people, especially when, without being aware of it, they slipped into spontaneous trance states.

Because of their trusting nature, relative gullibility, and inclination to accept uncritically the things they were told, the high eye rollers were often easy targets for slick salesmen, faith healers, cult leaders, and the like. "Compulsive compliance" was a feature of their psychological makeup. Conceivably, these trance-prone personalities could be talked into breaking the law in the naïve belief that they were doing the right thing.

Spiegel had then spoken of their opposite numbers: the low eye rollers, or Zeros and Ones, who seemed to have a built-in resistance to persuasion. They might well be obedient to someone in authority but only as a calculated choice, not because they had failed to consider their options or the consequences of their actions. If they carried out unlawful orders, it would be for reasons of their own, as a matter of "guileful compliance," and not because they naïvely believed what they were told. It was in their nature to be guarded and skeptical and never to lose touch with reality.

John Dean was curious to know where he stood on the scale of hypnotizability. Was he a Four or a Five with a Dionysian personality, as Spiegel had described it, or a Zero or a One with Apollonian traits? Or was he one of those in-between Odysseans with average trance capacity—the Twos and Threes—who made up most of the population?

During the symposium's lunch break, Dean approached Spiegel and asked him to examine his eye roll. Glad of the opportunity to see if his hunch about Dean's Apollonian nature was correct, Spiegel agreed and gave these directions:

"Look toward me. As you hold your head in that position, look up toward your eyebrows. Now toward the top of your head. As you continue to look upward, close your eyelids slowly. That's right, close. Close. Close." After a predictable bit of fluttering, Dean's eyelids finally closed. "All right," Spiegel said, "now open them."

The exercise took but a few seconds and the results were as expected. Dean's eyes had rolled only slightly, as if something within him had kept a tight rein on the tiny extraocular muscles to prevent the eyes from taking even a brief break from their customary sentry duty. In contrast, the eyes of a highly hypnotizable person would have rolled so easily during the initial upgaze that the irises would have almost disappeared beneath the upper eyelids. And then the irises would have vanished altogether as the eyelids began to close—which is the precise moment when the observer makes a mental note of the amount of sclera or white tissue visible between the irises and the lower eyelids.

"You're a One," Spiegel told Dean, meaning that he was

biologically incapable of producing the kind of easygoing eye roll that comes naturally to highly hypnotizable people. "You have some trance capacity but not much." In all likelihood, Dean could be hypnotized but he would always hold on to that large amount of control that the Apollonians cherish. He would not know the depths of trance that can be reached by the Odysseans and the still more trance-gifted Dionysians.

During the afternoon session of the symposium, Spiegel told the audience: "Mr. Dean's report of what he went through at Watergate—how he handled it, the way he negotiated his way out, how he was able to see his limited choices, and his internal need to make the choice the way he did—amounts to a textbook illustration of the man who has a low eye roll, who lives largely by his left hemisphere; a man who is always ready to critically scrutinize everything he does, even when he, in retrospect, realizes he is making an error." The title of Dean's Watergate book, after all, was *Blind Ambition*, not *Blind Obedience*.

Spiegel went on to say that if Dean were endowed with a high eye roll, which is the mark of a very different kind of brain wiring, he would probably have accepted the reasoning of his superiors and remained loyal to their efforts, however misguided. He would not have experienced so much inner turmoil about all the rights and wrongs.

"Yes," Dean agreed. "I was constantly analyzing what I was doing and why I was doing it, and I expect that's what led to my discomfort, because I wrestled with all these things and the anxiety was very heavy. But I did get out of it. I'm glad now that I wasn't a Five."

Poets have spoken of eyes as the windows of the soul. Philosophers like Emerson have described their universal language: "The eyes of men converse as much as their tongues." Researchers in sleep laboratories have discovered that our eyes move about rapidly beneath our lids when we dream. Our own observations tell us that surprise, delight, and fear, among other things, are commonly expressed by a widening or bulging of the eyes. When attempting to focus on a thought or remember something, most of us characteristically swivel our eyes to the right or left, or else we roll them up. The upward eye roll also serves as silent speech, signaling exasperation, resignation, and other feelings. (When grandfather launches into his favorite war story for the hundredth time, we raise our eyes to the ceiling—if we can—as a way of saying, "Oh, no, not again!")

The eye roll conveys still more serious messages. The writings of the ancient Greeks refer to upward eye movement in hysterical disturbances. Physicians have long been aware that convulsive behavior is likely to be accompanied by an eye roll, suggesting that normal controls over the eye muscles have been abandoned. Descriptions of so-called possession states and "out-of-body" experiences often speak of a rolling of the eyes.

The eye roll is a favorite staple of fiction writers as they seek to describe extremes of human conduct. More than a century ago, in "The Case of M. Valdemar," an imaginary account of an attempt to use mesmerism to forestall an invalid's imminent death, Edgar Allan Poe referred several times to the rolling of the patient's eyes as he went in and out of trance.

Charles Darwin, writing of love and religious faith in his classic work, *The Expressions of the Emotion in Man and Animals*, noted: "Devotion is chiefly expressed by the face being directed toward the heavens, with the eyeballs upturned. Sir C. [Charles] Bell remarks that, at the approach of sleep, or of a fainting-fit, or of death, the pupils are drawn upwards and inwards; and he believes that 'when we are wrapt in devotional feelings, and outward impressions are unheeded, the eyes are raised to an action neither taught nor acquired.' . . . With babies, whilst sucking their mother's breast, this movement of the eyeballs often gives to them an absurd appearance of ecstatic delight.''

Despite such instances of scholarly interest in upward eye movements, no one seemed to notice something that is perfectly obvious once attention is drawn to it: the fact that people differ strikingly in their ability to roll their eyes. Some do it with dramatic abandon; most do it to a lesser extent; some people cannot do it at all.

No theatergoer who witnessed Laurence Olivier in *Othello* can forget those great eyes rolling so far out of sight that nothing but gleaming white ovals could be seen on his dark face. There is all the difference in the world between the inhibited and almost imperceptible eye roll of a John Dean and the freewheeling eye movements of those who have a natural ability to let themselves go. Carol Burnett, as seen in television close-ups, is able to take an emotional moment and let her soaring eyes do the talking. Reggie Jackson's high eye rolls, captured in sports-page photographs, are consistent with his reputation as an exceptionally emotional and theatrical baseball player. Fernando Valenzuela of the Los Angeles Dodgers, who is momentarily in trance when he pitches, has made his eye roll a personal trademark.

Herbert Spiegel did not detect the differences in eye-roll behavior—and the significance of those differences—until he was well into his medical career. From then on, the eye roll as a biological sign of hypnotizability became the cornerstone of the whole new approach to hypnosis that he constructed.

The discovery of the Eye-Roll Sign was no "Eureka!" experience. "One day in 1963," Spiegel relates, "I got a call from a doctor I knew well. He said to me, 'Herb, I'm not asking you, I'm telling you! I've got a patient you must see right now. I'm sending her right over.' "

She was Mrs. Meyer, a stout, middle-aged housewife who had been afflicted for a year and a half with severe convulsive seizures. They occurred eight to twelve times a day. All the doctors who had examined her were stumped. She had been treated as an epileptic even though X rays and electroencephalograms revealed no sign of epilepsy or anything else that might provide an explanation.

Each of Mrs. Meyer's seizures lasted for fifteen to twenty minutes. She would fall to the floor, thrash about with her mouth open and her eyes rolled up, and then have no memory of what had happened. The seizures were frightening to witness. They seemed to have a life of their own. No intervention could cut them short. Anyone present during an attack felt compelled to hold her down or sit on her to keep her from hurting herself. The Meyer family was in turmoil. Her husband would rush home from work when called during a particularly bad episode. Her sons took turns staying at home so that she would not be left alone. Her doctors were intimidated by the violence of the seizures.

Spiegel's matter-of-fact approach was something new. "All right," he said to her at their first meeting, "let me see you do it. Show me a seizure." Though he did not then have the advantage of the Hypnotic Induction Profile, he suspected that she was highly hypnotizable and thought it likely that the convulsions were hysterical rather than organic. For one thing, instead of clenching her fists and tightening her mouth as an epileptic will during a convulsion, she extended her fingers and opened her mouth. In the absence of an organic explanation for the spasms, this strongly suggested to Spiegel "a profound trance experience in the service of some kind of psycho-pathological need." In short, hysteria.

Stating that the seizures came on without warning, Mrs. Meyer insisted that she could not start one by her-self. "I'll help you start it," Spiegel said. He guided her into trance. "Okay," he said, "let it happen." And it did. The convulsion was so powerful that she slipped out of her chair and began writhing on the floor. Finding that nothing he said could stop the seizure, Spiegel waited un-til it had run its course.

"This is great!" he exclaimed when she was back to normal. "Now I have something to show you." He told her that she had begun the seizure on her own. There-fore, it was something she could control. "What you can start, you can stop." By bringing on the seizures herself instead of waiting for them to happen, she could abbrevi-ate them. He was building on the fact that she already was exerting greater control than she realized. She had not, for example, ever been hurt during a convulsion even though it seemed so dangerous. She was like the typical somnambulist, or sleepwalker, who somehow manages to walk around obstacles and step through door-ways instead of crashing into walls even though deep in trance and seemingly far removed from the real world.

Spiegel's purpose was to add conscious control to un-conscious control. "The strategy," he explains, "was to have her produce a number of small, controlled seizures during the day so that it would not be necessary to have the big ones. There was something going on that we didn't know about. It seemed that the seizures were bound to happen, like an emotional charge that had to find an outlet. If it built up too much it got out of con-trol, so I taught her a self-hypnosis exercise as prevention. I said, 'If you feel it coming on, quickly do it on your own. That takes the wind out of the sails of the big ones.'

So it was partly preventive, partly therapeutic. She mastered it very quickly."

Mrs. Meyer became adept at putting herself into a trance by closing her eyes and raising a hand to her forehead, as if brushing away a lock of hair. This gesture was her signal to herself to bring on a seizure. She would then turn it off by counting backward from three to one. In time, she was able to reduce each convulsion to less than a minute so that it amounted to a ripple instead of a wave; more of a shudder than a seizure.

Learning self-control through self-hypnosis meant that Mrs. Meyer was no longer the cause of disruption at home and the object of pity and concern. Her personal life improved immeasurably. She could leave the house and go about without embarrassment.

"In those days," Spiegel recalls, "I was still influenced by my analytic training. I didn't imagine that a case with such a spectacular symptom could be handled in one or two sessions. I saw her for weekly sessions for a couple of months but I wouldn't do it today. Once you've identified hypnotizability in a patient and you show her that she has the capacity to control the symptom with self-hypnosis, then that's it. I would want the patient to keep me informed about her progress, but my approach would be a kind of respectful impatience: 'Get going. Don't depend on me. You're the one who's got the answer.' Psychoanalytically, of course, there must have been a gold mine of information that would help explain Mrs. Meyer's seizures but, typical of the Dionysians, she was not curious about the reasons. She had no interest in doing any digging. To her, this was just a nightmare that she wanted to be done with. My belief is that you don't go beyond the patient's curiosity. It's really an intrusion if you force exploration when a person isn't interested."

The case of Mrs. Meyer so intrigued Spiegel that he

made a teaching film of her convulsions and her ability to master them. "I watched that movie many times," he says, "and one day while I was looking at it again I was impressed by the way her eyes rolled way up during the seizures. It occurred to me that such mobile eyes might be special to highly hypnotizable people. Perhaps hypnotists had never noticed it because they were always asking people to close their eyes. I thought that maybe I should do the opposite and ask people to keep their eyes open so that I could see how far they could look up. Although I told myself that there couldn't be anything to this wild idea I decided to look into it anyway. That was on a Saturday. When my first patient came in Monday morning at nine o'clock I asked him to roll up his eyes and he couldn't. He also couldn't be hypnotized. He was a paranoid, obsessive personality, and we know now that such a person is not hypnotizable. Anyway, it was obvious that the ability to roll one's eyes was not universal.

"As you might imagine, I spent the next year staring at eyes and doing informal measurements. The upgaze was important because if it was high you could expect trance capacity to be high, but I learned that I should ask people to slowly close the eyes while holding the upgaze. You would see the eye roll at its best. That was the time to measure. When we got to the point where we could predict with considerable accuracy whether a patient could be hypnotized, and to what extent, we started doing very systematic measurements that eventually numbered in the thousands.

"Also, while examining eye rolls, I started looking for other signs of hypnotic ability. Arm levitation, for example. In trance, the arm of a person with a high eye roll would start rising at the mere suggestion that the hand was so light that it would float in the air. With other people, you had to give more concrete suggestions, like saying that a balloon attached to the hand is helping it rise. I also found that people differed in the feeling of control that they had in one arm as opposed to the other when there was levitation. We could match these differences with their eye-roll scores. That's how the idea of the Hypnotic Induction Profile emerged. Once I saw that hypnosis had nothing to do with sleep and that the eye roll was an important factor, it came to me that hypnosis was a way of paying attention—*really* paying attention. I got the idea that hypnosis was the exact opposite of sleep: a state of intense, alert concentration. Instead of being in some kind of foggy, sleepy condition, the hypnotized person was really being super-alert, super-attentive. And I thought: Well, hell, maybe this is something that we can measure. Maybe this is how a doctor can find out beforehand how a patient will take to hypnosis."

For his eye-roll measurement, Spiegel devised a zero-to-four scale for the amount of white space between the iris and the lower eyelid as seen just before the subject, while still looking all the way up, closes his or her eyes. Most people were in the one-to-three range, and their modest to impressive eye rolls were matched by modest to impressive trance states *unless* there was some kind of psychological interference with a person's ability to express his natural trance capacity. The highest score, four, was given to those individuals whose eyes rotated out of sight. Such high rollers were the very people who, if not impaired in their ability to focus their minds, demonstrated trance in its deepest and most dramatic forms. Further testing of the "Fours" would reveal which of them were so extraordinarily hypnotizable that they deserved to be considered "Fives."

Spiegel came upon more than he had bargained for in his research effort. In a nice example of serendipity, he found that the eye roll not only revealed a person's biolog-

EYE-ROLL SIGN FOR HYPNOTIZABILITY

	Score
	0
	1
	2
	3
	4

ical gift for trance but, when juxtaposed with information about that person's actual expression of his trance talent, provided a strong signal about mental intactness or nonintactness. About a quarter of the people tested were unable to focus their minds well enough to use the trance capacity that they possessed. Thus the Eye-Roll Sign, as it is now known in medical literature, must be seen as only a very rough indicator of how any given individual will respond when a trance induction is attempted. It can, however, be taken as a reliable tipoff of hypnotic responsivity among the three quarters of the population who are mentally sound. In turn, to use Spiegel's words, "hypnotic capacity implies reasonably good, nonpsychotic, mental health."

The alert reader will notice that Spiegel appears to be saying that there is something wrong with the mental functioning of about a quarter of the population. That is exactly what he is saying, but he is not the first to come to such a conclusion. The publication in 1962 of *Mental Health in the Metropolis: The Midtown Manhattan Study* made public the results of a remarkably comprehensive and now-classic survey of mental health conducted several years earlier in a major area of New York City. The team of Cornell University researchers, directed by a noted psychiatrist, Dr. Leo Srole, found that nearly 25 percent of the Manhattan residents who were interviewed suffered from a variety of mild-to-serious emotional problems. A less well-known survey conducted at about the same time in Stirling County, Nova Scotia, by Cornell researchers found that about a third of the residents suffered from emotional impairment.

What is new in Spiegel's work is the finding that an individual's inability to go into hypnosis when he has the biological ability to do so (as revealed by the eye roll) is a fairly accurate predictor of mental dysfunction. As the following chapter describes, the combination of the eye-roll measurement and data about a person's actual trance experience can give a doctor a strong signal about mental health and the likely response to various treatment strategies.

Spiegel's clinical research into the significance of the eye roll yielded something else: the revelation that eye-roll and trance-capacity measurements can speak volumes about who we are as personalities.

"I couldn't believe it at first," Spiegel says. "Everything I found went against my training." Like a great many psychiatrists, he had viewed individual personality as more the product of upbringing and circumstances than genetic coding. "But then I came to see that hypnosis is a capacity for attentive, receptive concentration that is inherent in a person, and that whatever it is in the brain that governs this capacity governs the degree of eye roll. As a result, I've made a 180-degree shift. Today I believe that the major determination of who we are as people is pretty much decided when the sperm meets the egg."

An individual's eye roll, however mobile it may be, is essentially stable and permanent just as one's capacity for hypnosis is essentially stable and permanent. Though Spiegel's research indicates that there may be a slight reduction in the amount of eye roll, as in hypnotic ability, over the course of a lifetime, the change is so gradual that a youth who scores as a Three, for example, can be expected to remain a Three or close to it most of his life. In his old age he very likely would score as a Two. Children take to hypnosis more readily than adults just as they give freer rein to their imaginations than adults, but they too vary in trance capacity.

"On the whole, we remain the hypnotic people we were programmed to be," Spiegel says. "A person with a low eye roll is never going to have a high eye roll, and vice versa." Practice would not give a Dean the soaring eye roll of an Olivier.

Spiegel recalls an exception that proves the rule, however. "There was a doctor who took the course a few years ago who had a high eye roll, indicating that he was a Four. But when we did further testing with the Profile, we found that his arm levitation and other features of the test put him on the low side of the hypnotizability scale. We were baffled as to why an apparently mentally intact Apollonian should have a Dionysian eye roll. After we did a lot of speculating he came up with an anecdote about himself. It seems that when he was a child he entered a contest to see who could come closest to imitating Ben Turpin, the movie comedian whose eyes revolved in all directions. He practiced rolling his eyes every day and ended up winning the contest. That led us to believe that in the developmental years people could get artificial movements of their eye muscles if they practiced enough. But I don't think they could do it so well as adults."

In his own psychiatric work in California, David Spiegel routinely checks out a patient's eye roll—and conducts the rest of the Hypnotic Induction Profile—as a screening device. "I test for hypnotizability just as you test other aspects of a person's mental functioning. It is tremendously helpful in determining a patient's capacities and resources for treatment and also for ruling in or ruling out certain types of disorders. We have found, for example, that there are some patients who have been diagnosed as schizophrenic but who show you a very high eye roll. When you do further testing you discover that they are really highly hypnotizable people who are very compliant and very quick to pick up cues in the surroundings of a mental institution—and who, in effect, have learned to behave as schizophrenics."

There was a time, however, when David was skeptical about the whole idea of the eye roll as a valid sign that could give a doctor useful information about his patient.

"That was true until the day I realized that my father had come up with something that really worked. I was a third-year medical student at Harvard and he had been invited to come up to Boston to do grand rounds at Beth Israel Hospital. I was present along with Fred Frankel, a professor of psychiatry, and other doctors, when he demonstrated the Profile test, beginning with the eye roll.

"They brought in two student nurses as volunteers. He looked at their eye rolls and he predicted how they would perform. And he was exactly wrong in both cases. Since the first girl had practically no eye roll he figured she would be a poor hypnotic subject but when he did the rest of the Profile she proved to be high in trance capacity. The second girl had a high eye roll but he couldn't hypnotize her. I could only think: Well, Pop, too bad; there goes that theory; it's been nice knowing you.

"But he has always said that the eye roll is not a perfect indicator—just a pretty good indicator—of how someone will perform in hypnosis. You have to do the full Profile test to get the whole story. In this case, something I thought was really amazing happened after he saw that the Eye-Roll Sign was misleading. He asked the first girl whether she had ever had eye-muscle surgery. 'Oh, yes,' she said. 'I had a squint when I was a little girl and they shortened my eye muscles.' That explained why her eye roll didn't match her trance capacity. Dr. Frankel was so impressed with this that he signed up for the next course at Columbia. Today he runs the Clinic for Therapeutic Hypnosis at Beth Israel.

"As for the other girl, we discovered that she was a barbiturate addict. She had a high eye roll and would normally be highly hypnotizable, but because she was constantly stoned on barbiturates she couldn't concentrate well enough to go into trance."

9

THE PROFILE

He who wishes to show us a truth should place us in a situation where we will discover it for ourselves.

—Ortega y Gasset,
Meditations on Quixote

For several years prior to his discovery of the eye roll, Dr. Spiegel was troubled by the fact that physicians using hypnosis did so more by guesswork and gut feelings than by any kind of disciplined, scientific method.

"Most of them weren't concerned about assessing trance capacity," he says, "or varying their treatment according to the hypnotizability of their patients. They simply assumed that everybody was hypnotizable and that inducing trance depended solely on the power or skill of the hypnotist. As you can imagine, this led to situations where the doctor would knock himself out trying to hypnotize someone who simply could not be hypnotized. Some patients would become so tired or annoyed by the whole business that they would pretend to be in a trance. But even those doctors who understood that people varied greatly in their hypnotic ability had no way of accurately monitoring the trance performances of their patients and no way of comparing notes with other doctors. Everything was at an anecdotal level."

Spiegel felt then that medical hypnosis was not likely

to have much of a future until doctors who were not seat-of-the-pants therapists could think of it, like the rest of medicine, as a science as well as an art. Clearly needed was a brief but accurate test for trance capacity that would fit into the busy routine of a clinic and give a doctor not just a basis for deciding whether to try hypnosis but some idea of the nature of the trance that his patient might achieve. Treatment strategy would be selected to match the extent of trance capacity. Spiegel's interest in devising such a test was stimulated by some questions raised by one of the physicians he had trained in hypnosis.

"When the Columbia course first began," he relates, "I spent a lot of time showing the doctors a variety of traditional hypnotic-induction techniques—everything from eye fixation and arm paralysis to body swaying and fixing on a moving object or flashing light. I was trying to say that if you know the principles, it doesn't matter what procedure you use. Just take one that you feel comfortable with and do it. And, of course, that's the way it should be. The ceremony for inducing hypnosis doesn't matter; what counts is what you do with the trance state once you've got it. But then this doctor came up to me and said, 'This is a fascinating course, but how do you *really* induce a trance state?' I was ready to fall to the floor. I couldn't believe it. I said, 'What do you think we've been doing here with all these demonstrations?' And he said that, yes, the people seemed to go into trance but how did I know they were *really* in trance? And he was right! We didn't have a test to prove that the hypnosis was genuine. And even if it was genuine, we couldn't say with any precision what kind of trance we were dealing with.

"I thought how great it would be if we had some standards for the trance state so that everyone looking at the same thing would be able to agree that a subject not only is capable of the trance experience but actually goes into trance. Then when I got onto the eye roll by watching the Meyer film, and later on tied that to arm levitation, a more conventional factor of hypnosis, we were on our way to producing a practical clinical test for hypnotic capacity that any doctor could use with any patient."

Spiegel's Hypnotic Induction Profile was published as a clinical manual in 1968 and introduced to members of the American Society of Clinical Hypnosis at their 1970 annual conference. Largely because hundreds of practitioners in the last decade have been trained in the HIP procedure at the Columbia course, the Profile is now well established nationwide among doctors who wish to give a more scientific underpinning to their use of hypnosis. Many more clinicians who are less interested in assessing hypnotizability turn to the Eye-Roll Sign alone to get a quick clue about a patient's trance potential while simultaneously letting the eye roll serve as the start of a trance induction.

Several tests for hypnotic responsivity, principally the Stanford Hypnotic Susceptibility Scales, preceded Spiegel's Profile. They had been devised and refined in university laboratories in the 1950s and 1960s and had proved to be invaluable to investigators of hypnotic phenomena. Psychologists, behavioral researchers, and others had used them to make hypnosis more of a scientific discipline.

Unfortunately, the tests employed by academic experimenters were neither practical nor appropriate in a clinical setting. They had not been designed for medical hypnosis. The Stanford Scales, for example, took about an hour to administer and contained features that might well tire, confuse, and even offend a patient who had gone to the doctor for relief from a symptom, not to be a subject in a research project.

Spiegel was troubled by the "go to sleep" and "wake up" terminology of the established tests because his clinical experience had persuaded him that hypnosis was anything but sleep. He disputed the use of the term "hypnotic susceptibility" because it implied a weakness. He preferred describing hypnosis more positively as an expression of an individual's capacity to focus his mind and become extraordinarily alert and imaginative.

Spiegel also questioned the soundness (as well as the usefulness to a clinician) of data from tests that were usually given to university students, often paid volunteers, as opposed to a patient population of all ages and backgrounds, varying greatly in physical and mental health. Such tests were too remote from the realities of a doctor's office where the patient's illness, his desire for a remedy, and the quality of his rapport with the physician could all affect the trance experience. Hypnosis, as Spiegel saw it, was a marriage of biological and psychological influences, and he thought it vital in measuring hypnotizability to account for them.

The Hypnotic Induction Profile test teaches as it measures. For the typical patient, it is a learning experience, not just a procedure to give the doctor information about his hypnotizability. He is introduced to formal hypnosis for the first time and sees for himself what it is and what it is not. Unless he lacks all trance capacity, he discovers that he has a gift for an altered state of consciousness that he had not realized. This relaxing ritual, which takes only five to ten minutes (and does not have to be repeated in any future visit to the doctor), prepares the patient for self-hypnosis. Now that he knows the simple steps for shifting into the trance state, he can do it on his own. He can solo.

The doctor administering the HIP test—both guiding the patient through hypnosis and marking on a score sheet the way the patient enters, experiences, and exits the trance state—is like a flying instructor: He not only gives directions to a novice pilot who is at the controls for the first time but takes notes on the manner of the take-off, flight, and landing. The resulting Profile score, Spiegel explains, "is a statement of the relationship between a person's potential for trance as revealed by the eye roll and his ability to experience and maintain it." A score sheet may be a puzzle to anyone unfamiliar with the symbols, but to the doctor it is a graphic depiction of the patient's trance capacity that he can use to select a treatment strategy.

In the typical administration of the test, the doctor, after seeing to it that his patient is comfortably seated in an armchair, begins by asking him to do an eye roll. He records the result according to a zero-to-four scale. Instead of telling the patient to open his eyes again, as Spiegel did after checking John Dean's eye roll, the doctor uses the eye roll to begin the trance induction. He asks the patient to take a deep breath and hold it. "Now exhale," he continues. "Let your eyes relax while keeping the lids closed, and let your body float. Imagine a feeling of floating."

Though the patient at this stage is probably well into hypnosis, he might not think so because he continues to be conscious of where he is and what he is doing. His mind is focused both on the doctor's voice and on the feeling of floating. (Spiegel points out to the patient after the test: "As you see, hypnosis is not sleep. It's not blacking out. It's a method of concentration and a double awareness. You're here and beside yourself at the same time. You were paying attention to me at the same time that you were aware of new sensations.")

The test continues when the doctor states: "I am going to stroke the middle finger of your left hand. After I do, you will develop movement sensations in that finger. Then the movements will spread, causing your left hand to feel light and buoyant, and you will let it float upward. Ready?"

He strokes the finger. For some, the highly hypnotizable, there is immediate arm levitation. For the less hypnotizable, the arm will float upward, if at all, only after further suggestions and perhaps even an instruction to "let your hand be a balloon."

The doctor makes a note of the levitation score (zero to four) and then moves on to a series of instructions for further assessment of hypnotic responsivity. He tells the patient that his left arm will remain in its upright position even after he receives a signal to open his eyes. In fact, the doctor says, "When your eyes are open, even when I put your hand down, it will float right back up to where it is now. You will find something amusing about this sensation. Later, when I touch your left elbow, your usual sensation and control will return. In the future, each time you give yourself the signal for self-hypnosis, at the count of one your eyes will roll upward and by the count of three your eyelids will close and you will feel in a relaxed trance state. Each time you will find the experience easier and easier. Now I am going to count backward. At two, your eyes will again roll upward with your eyelids closed. At one, let them open very slowly. Ready? Three. Two. With your eyelids closed, roll up your eyes. And one, let them open slowly."

These are the instructions for ending the formal trance ceremony. Seemingly, the patient, his eyes now open, is out of trance. Actually, Spiegel says, he is in a postceremonial trance state because a part of his mind is still focused on something told him during the formal trance: that his left arm will remain upright and will even float again when the doctor pulls his hand down. This state of mind can be thought of as a kind of lingering double awareness. Now that the trance appears to be over, the person is back to the "real world" (which he never completely left), yet some part of his mind is still in hypnosis. The phenomenon is something like the afterglow that a theatergoer may feel for a while after the curtain comes down on a play that has completely caught his imagination. Traditionally, hypnosis experts have called it "posthypnotic" but Spiegel prefers the term "postceremonial," arguing that hypnosis is still in progress despite the completion of the trance ceremony.

The patient's reactions at this stage of the test are scored. The doctor observes whether his left arm stays aloft after he opens his eyes. And whether it floats upward once again after the hand is pulled down. Finally, the patient is asked to raise and lower his right arm. He is given the question: "Are you aware of any difference in your sense of control in one arm going up, compared to the other?"

In most instances, the patient reports that his left arm, which can be thought of as the hypnotized arm, not only feels lighter than the right arm but seems to have a mind of its own. This is marked on the score sheet as another positive sign of his ability to live up to his trance potential. Spiegel sees the control differential as the key item of the Profile test. "It reveals integrated concentration. The subject is not instructed beforehand to feel this difference. It is *discovered* in this context, and the discovery itself contributes to the patient's understanding of hypnosis."

The test comes to an end, and so does the trance state, when the doctor touches the patient's left elbow, as he earlier said he would. This is the "cutoff" signal. Usual sensation and control are restored. The doctor now has the information he needs on the patient's suitability for medical hypnosis. For most people, the test results show that performance during hypnosis matches the promise of the eye roll. It can be said of them that the eye roll tells the whole story because the rest of the test features simply fall in line with the eye-roll measurement. Thus a patient with an eye roll of three proves to have the responses of a Three during trance.

Because of the existence of the Hypnotic Induction Profile, it is now clearer than ever not just that people differ widely in their biological talent for hypnosis but that there are crucial differences in their ability to employ the talent they have. For medical hypnosis, this is an all-important distinction.

Profile research confirms the findings of a number of experimental hypnotists, using the Stanford Scales in academic settings, that there is a small percentage of people at one extreme who seem to be completely devoid of hypnotic talent and a small percentage at the other extreme who are supremely suited to the trance state. As for those in between, they are the great majority who reveal meager to major capacity for hypnosis.

Unlike the laboratory measurements, however, the Profile's purpose is not to detect fine gradations of hypnotic responsivity in a succession of test subjects. Its purpose is to determine in a clinical setting whether an individual seeking medical help is likely to respond well to hypnosis as a treatment modality. The degree of trance capacity revealed by the test suggests the best treatment strategy to employ. An approach that is tailored for the talent and personality of a Dionysian might not work at all with an Apollonian or an Odyssean.

Clinicians who use the Profile are concerned with the individual patient, not with producing statistics about the distribution of hypnotic ability in the population. If there are many patients, however, and their Profile scores are eventually examined, as Spiegel has done, interesting patterns of hypnotizability can be seen.

Seventy percent of the people tested by Spiegel—and by others involved in Profile-based research—are hypnotizable. They have no difficulty expressing their trance talent to the full.

Twenty-five percent are not hypnotizable even though they have a biological capacity for hypnosis. Something interferes with the full expression of their trance ability.

Finally, 5 percent are not hypnotizable because they lack the means. Trance ability is not part of their makeup.

Obviously, those in the great majority—the hypnotizable 70 percent—are prime candidates for medical hypnosis. Not only do their eye rolls reveal a built-in potential for trance, but they succeed in fully utilizing that potential. Spiegel describes their individual Profiles as "intact" because the matching of promise (the eye-roll score) and performance (the full Profile score) is a sign of psychological integration. In other words, the Intacts, as he calls them, come equipped with the brain wiring for hypnosis and have no problem putting it into operation.

Among the Intacts, those with the least trance capacity are the Ones. Some traditional hypnotists might suppose that the Ones are not hypnotizable because they do not go deeply into trance. But Spiegel has demonstrated that many people who seem to have little or no talent for hypnosis are still capable of therapeutically useful trance states.

The majority of the Intacts are mid-range—Twos and Threes. Those with the highest Profile scores are the Fours. Some Fours prove in further testing to be capable of such profound trance experiences (age regression, for one thing) that they are elevated to Fives. These hypnotic superstars make up 5 percent of the adult population.

(People who fall in between the scale gradations are identified as One-Twos, Two-Threes, and Three-Fours.)

The Fives who stand at one end of the hypnotizability
scale because of their superior trance talent are balanced
by about as many individuals at the other end who have
no trance talent at all. They are the Zeros: the 5 percent
who are not hypnotizable because they lack the means.
There is no psychological impediment to their expression
of trance talent because there is no talent to express. The
no-hypnosis message of their eye rolls is confirmed by the
rest of the test.

(It is noteworthy, however, that many Zeros as they
appear in a doctor's office are so motivated—either for the
hypnotic experience or clinical treatment, or both—that
signs of trance turn up in the test. Some arm levitation
may be seen. Sheer desire, it seems, propels them into a
facsimile of the trance state and the alert clinician may
well be able to use it in therapy. Spiegel calls them Special
Zeros.)

The 25 percent who have a biological capacity for
trance and yet cannot be hypnotized, at least sufficiently
for the purposes of medical hypnosis, are described as
Nonintacts. Various mild-to-serious mental disturbances
get in the way as they try to express their trance talent.
Performance fails to match potential. A Nonintact with a
high eye roll is like a ballplayer who has all the physical
gifts for hitting home runs but who can do nothing at bat
but strike out or hit pop flies. As much as these people
may wish to enter the trance state and use it as others do,
they have great difficulty focusing their minds and maintaining concentration.

A typical Nonintact Profile score sheet shows a positive
eye roll, anything from one to four; but everything else is
zero. The subject does not respond to arm-levitation suggestions, feels no difference of control in one arm as op-

posed to the other, and, overall, gives no sign of being in a hypnotic state.

The Nonintacts who completely fail to go into trance are called Decrements by Spiegel because of their decrement or diminished-capacity Profiles. Those who partially match the promise of their eye rolls are known as Softs because theirs is a softer fall from potential.

In *Trance and Treatment*, the Spiegels attempt to explain why a substantial number of people fall below the biological baseline revealed by their eye rolls and fail to reach their trance potential: "For schizophrenics, this may be due to the fragmentation of attention and concentration—their distractibility and loose associations. For those with paranoid or obsessional character disorders, the trance experience may arouse too much anxiety, suspicion, and fears about the operator controlling the patient. Sociopaths may fear that the hypnotic situation makes them too vulnerable to manipulation, a projection of their own style of dealing with others. Those with serious depressions may be so narcissistically withdrawn and devoid of energy that they cannot attend to the input signals. Manics, on the other hand, may be so energized and grandiose that they disdain following the instructions which are part of the trance induction."

For the busy clinician, it is a blessing to be able to identify quickly those patients—the seven out of every ten—who can be expected to go into trance without difficulty and fully utilize their hypnotic capacity. The Profile scores even tell him which of his hypnotizable patients are so strongly motivated that they actually go beyond their trance potential during hypnosis. They are called Special Intacts.

A patient is not rejected for treatment, of course, if testing indicates a lack of basic hypnotic capacity or an interference with a natural gift for trance. Hypnosis, after all, can give leverage to therapy but it is not itself therapy. The patient still has a problem that deserves treatment even if there is not to be the extra thrust that the trance state can provide.

Dr. Spiegel's conclusions about the range of hypnotizability in the adult population are based on an impressive body of data. There are, first of all, the very detailed analyses that have been made by Spiegel and his research staff of the Profile scores of 4,621 patients seen and tested in his office between 1969 and 1976. In every case, the administration of the Profile was done as a routine clinical procedure, much as a family doctor might wish to check the pulse and blood pressure of each new patient. More than half of Spiegel's patients came for stop-smoking treatment. Most of the others complained of being overweight or else presented the kind of problems that lend themselves to short-term psychotherapy.

Since 1976, Spiegel has obtained Profiles from more than five thousand additional patients. He has also tested many other people: doctors attending the Columbia course; volunteers who come forward when he lectures at universities and scientific conferences; witnesses and suspects when he is asked to give expert testimony in criminal cases. He has been able to match his own results with the hundreds of Profiles gathered by David Spiegel in California, by Barbara DeBetz in her own New York practice, and by those clinicians and researchers—especially Edward J. Frischholz of Columbia University—who have been involved in this continuing study of hypnotizability.

Because of such an exceptionally large population sampling, and because it has been possible—with the aid of computers—to determine the influence of sex, age, intelligence, educational levels, and other factors on hypnotic responsivity, Spiegel is on solid ground when he speaks about the trance differences and the trance styles of people in general. As mentioned in earlier chapters, he is able to say that, as hypnotic beings, men and women are much the same; that trance capacity among adults, although changing little over a lifetime, is at its peak in the early years; and that greater intelligence (as measured by standard tests) and higher levels of education go with higher Profile scores. "One of the things we are surest about after seeing plenty of studies," Spiegel says, "is that we don't get hypnotizability at the bottom of the IQ scale."

Something else that he feels increasingly sure about is that the capacity for hypnosis is a sign of preference for right-hemispheric functioning. The more hypnotizable a person is, it seems, the more likely it is that he deals with the world primarily through the right side of his brain. Spiegel's confidence that hypnotic ability is preeminently genetic—more a matter of nature than nurture—has been enhanced with virtually every announcement of discoveries by investigators of brain functioning. The work of Dr. Roger W. Sperry, a winner of the 1981 Nobel Prize for medicine, and other pioneers in split-brain research have revealed that we process the information of our senses in very different ways. Each hemisphere has its own cognitive style. The left brain is on the job when we try to understand the words of a newspaper article or a political speech; the right brain pretty much takes over when we lean back and enjoy beautiful music.

The left hemisphere is verbal, mathematical, and analytical as it devours facts and figures and takes charge of speech, writing, and other symbolic functions. We reason and explain ourselves with the left brain. In contrast, the right hemisphere is the seat of our more subjective and emotional selves. It is in charge of such nonverbal functions as spatial perception, artistic expression, imagery, and analogical thinking. Creativity seems to spring more from the right than from the left. The left brain is said to function at a higher level of arousal. It is tense, so to speak, in comparison to the more relaxed right brain. A person who produces alpha waves when his brain is hooked up to a machine for electroencephalograph measurements is understood to be dwelling almost exclusively in his right hemisphere—which is exactly where a mystic or meditator or Indian yogi chooses to be. Hypnotically talented people deliver more alpha waves.

Inasmuch as hypnosis appears to be a matter of shifting into the right-brain mode while leaving the left brain in neutral, it is not surprising that people who favor the right brain take to hypnosis and experience it more deeply than others. Those who have a natural preference for left-brain functioning find it more difficult to switch over to the right-brain mode that is required for the trance state. Most people, it seems, oscillate between the two hemispheres—now favoring the right, now favoring the left.

If we are observant enough, we can pick up clues about hemispheric leanings in the way most people—but not all people—move their eyes and their hands. These movements also disclose the likely hypnotic ranking of the individuals. Split-brain researchers tell us, for example, that most people can be classified as either "right-lookers" or "left-lookers." A person who is asked a question that requires some thought is likely to move his eyes either to the right or to the left as he reflects on the answer. He characteristically shifts his eyes in one direction and not the other. Broadly speaking, the right-looker favors his *left* hemisphere while the left-looker favors his *right* hemisphere. There is evidence that right-lookers are lower in trance talent. They reveal lower eye rolls and have more Apollonian traits than the left-lookers who are more hypnotizable, display higher eye rolls, and have more Dionysian personality features.

Dr. Spiegel has taken a particular interest in the hand clasp as a measure of hemispheric preference because it correlates well with hypnotizability as measured by the Profile. He has found that it is possible to look at the way a person clasps his hands—and even the way he claps his hands—and get a reasonably accurate preview of that person's trance possibilities.

It works this way: In most cases, if an individual is asked to hold his hands in front of his chest and to interlock the fingers, he will characteristically put the thumb and fingers of one hand on top of the thumb and corresponding fingers of the other hand. Most people find it awkward doing it any other way; it feels almost as strange as eating with the "wrong" hand. A "dominant clasp" is revealed if a right-handed person puts his right thumb on top or if a left-hander places his left hand on top. A dominant clasp indicates a greater reliance on the left hemisphere: the side of the brain that has the least to do with hypnosis.

After directing a formal study of 946 patients several years ago and observing the hand clasps of thousands of other people since then, Spiegel feels safe in saying that a dominant clasp is a strong indicator that the person is on the low side of the hypnotizability scale and will display various Apollonian features. In turn, but not so strongly, a nondominant clasp (when a right-hander puts his left thumb on top or a left-hander puts his right thumb on top) suggests medium to high hypnotizability.

"What's messing up the data," Spiegel says, "is that something like 20 percent of the population have mixed dominance. When that factor is eliminated, then the hand clasp is a pretty good signpost if you're wondering about a person's hypnotic qualities. The same can be said for the way people applaud. If a right-handed person claps his hands by bringing the right hand down on the left, then he probably has a low eye roll. The same is true for the left hander if his left hand is dominant when he applauds. In contrast, if you see a right-hander applauding by putting his nondominant hand, the left, on top—or if a left-hander puts the right hand on top—the chances are that he is mid-range or high in trance capacity."

For the astute clinician, any information about a patient's hemispheric preference and his hypnotic nature is good information. Different thinking styles call for different treatment strategies. As Spiegel says, the doctor will be in a position to "speak the patient's language."

10

APOLLONIANS–ODYSSEANS– DIONYSIANS

Tell me where is fancy bred . . .
Or in the heart or in the head?
—SHAKESPEARE, *The Merchant
of Venice*

"Several years ago," Dr. Spiegel relates, "I was invited to give a lecture to a group of high-powered executives who were at a retreat organized by the Columbia business school. They had been together for a month, attending a series of seminars on the theme of reexamining the issues that come before the top people in business.

"At that time I was just beginning to correlate eye rolls and personality styles. I talked to them about hypnosis and the characteristics of people who were low, mid-range, and high in trance capacity. I explained why I called them Apollonians, Odysseans, and Dionysians, and why an appreciation of their differing traits was important to the therapist. I said that a patient's eye roll provides a strong signal about his basic personality as well as his hypnotic capacity. Also that measuring an eye roll takes only seconds because it is merely a matter of knowing what to look for. The executives were really intrigued by all this. There were more than two dozen of them, mostly men, and they all volunteered to have their eye rolls examined.

"Given the nature of the business world, where there is such a premium on being shrewd and tough and analytical, I expected that most of them would be on the low side, and that's how it turned out. Everyone was a Two or under. Except for one man. He was a Three-Four, the only Dionysian. I found out later that he was the one they always turned to as a mediator when there was a dispute—the one person that everyone could relate to. They even elected him Mr. Congeniality at the end of the retreat.

"This man agreed that he had most of the attributes that I listed for the Dionysians. Basically, he was a sensitive, sympathetic, trusting person who was more likely to react to events with his heart than his head. The other executives asked him: If you're such an easygoing pussycat, how can you make all these tough business decisions and keep people from taking advantage of you? He told them that he now realized how he had been able to survive as a Dionysian in the Apollonian world of business. He said that when he was a college student, his rich uncle, a successful businessman, had warned him, 'If you want to make it in this world, you'd better learn to be an S.O.B. like me.' So he modeled himself after his uncle and put on such a performance as a hardheaded executive that he sometimes fantasized about his children coming to the office and not recognizing him. 'I'm a different person with my family,' he said, 'because when I go home from work I leave my Apollonian cloak in the office.'

"In other words, he was a closet Dionysian. He was able to play the role of a corporation big shot because highly hypnotizable people are chameleons. They can be almost anything."

Spiegel first began to link trance capacity to personality traits in the late 1960s when he observed that the most hypnotizable of his patients—the Fours and Fives—had a number of characteristics in common and that, when troubled, they encountered distinctive psychological problems. The propensities of extremely trance-talented people were stunningly revealed in hypnosis, of course. More importantly, they were evident in their customary behavior and life-style, and their way of dealing with people and events.

There was something credulous and guileless about highly hypnotizable individuals, Spiegel noticed. They had rich imaginations. They tended to act on their feelings more often than on logic or analysis. Instead of insisting on facts and figures, as many people do, they relied on their intuition. They trusted their hunches and followed their emotions. As their mobile eyes and expressive faces suggested, they tended to be open, impulsive, empathetic, and much inclined to take a hopeful, anything-is-possible outlook on life. It seemed to be in their nature to accept the control of others in many instances—rather than to insist on being in charge themselves. They almost seemed to be saying: Tell me what to believe and I'll believe it. In Spiegel's experience, the compliance of highly hypnotizable patients who were psychologically disturbed was often so great that it suggested a sense of inferiority: Who am I to know anything about this, compared to the person who is directing me?

After accumulating the Profile scores of more than four thousand patients of varying hypnotic abilities, Spiegel set down his conclusions about the trance-state extremists in a remarkable paper that was published in *The International Journal of Clinical and Experimental Hypnosis* in 1974. Many efforts had been made in hypnosis research to identify the special traits of exceptional trance subjects, but little had been achieved. There was no agreement among the experts about the personalities of either the hypnotic virtuoso or the individual who could not be hypnotized at all. Spiegel's paper was a revelation.

He called it "The Grade 5 Syndrome: The Highly Hypnotizable Person." He was careful to point out, however, that the features that are most obvious in the Fives are not exclusive to this group. "They appear to taper off as trance capacity decreases to the three level." Although the Fives account for only 5 percent of the population, their attributes, he says, "show up on a more or less basis in perhaps 20 to 25 percent of all people."

According to Spiegel, the Fives, in addition to their high eye rolls, their high-intact Profiles, and their propensity for spontaneous trance experiences, are distinguishable for their way of adopting "a naïve posture of trust" in relation to many if not all people in their environment. They "exude an intense, beguilingly innocent expectation of support from others." Indeed, "this incredibly demanding faith or trust goes beyond reasonable limits." The Fives display an absence of cynicism. They are prone to suspend critical judgment. They take things on faith instead of scrutinizing them for faults or hidden meanings. They exhibit "a willingness to replace, if necessary, old premises and beliefs with new ones without the usual cognitive screenings of the Ones, Twos, or the Zeroes."

The Fives can get themselves into trouble, Spiegel notes, by "looking at a simple proposal as a demand." He tells of a young New Yorker who had been suffering with a general despair about life for some time. "He went from doctor to doctor, and eventually consulted a well-known neurologist. This doctor was well informed about the patient's family background. He knew that the wealthy parents were obsessively self-preoccupied, and was aware as well that if the young man continued to live at home the outlook was bleak. During their second session, in an effort to arouse him, the doctor blurted out: 'John, why don't you go to Alaska and get away from it all? Start all over again.' When the patient left, he felt mildly dazed and profoundly reluctant to return home. Instead, he drove to a travel agent, where he obtained railway and airline schedules of trips to the West Coast. He kept thinking about Alaska, while at the same time telling himself that it was silly. Two days later, he flew to Alaska. There he occupied himself with hunting trips and guided tours of the state, but after a few months he realized the absurdity of what he was doing and returned to New York. He had taken the neurologist's metaphorical suggestion and acted upon it as if it were a literal command."

Such extreme suggestibility, when coupled with gullibility and a naïve trust in others, can make the highly hypnotizable personality vulnerable to deception. At the extreme, if told during trance to take a gun and kill someone, he almost surely would not carry out the instruction if his moral code held that murder was wrong. But what if the subject had first been told that a certain individual was a terrorist who must be stopped before he assassinated the President, and that it was his patriotic duty to take the gun, act like a soldier in combat, and kill the enemy? Under such conditions, the person conceivably might carry out the instructions. In other words, the idea of a "Manchurian Candidate" who is programmed to kill by a combination of drugs and hypnotic techniques, as in Richard Condon's 1959 novel, is not, in Spiegel's opinion, entirely implausible.

The personality traits that can get the Fives into trouble are also the qualities that are essential to the creative arts and scientific breakthroughs. "There is something awesome," Spiegel says, "about the ability of a highly hypnotizable person to convert these features into assets rather than liabilities. For example, a scientific investigator, to make discoveries, has to be wide open to new ideas and take an almost childlike approach to possibilities and new connections. Someone lower in trance ability is likely to be too critical of a new idea because it does not fit in with the old criteria—like the French fighting World War II with World War I tactics. The readiness of the Fives to replace old ideas with new ideas is a great advantage."

Related to this is the tendency of the Fives to affiliate with concrete events—to identify with here-and-now reality. They have an almost magnetic attraction to the immediate occurrence and an almost irresistible urge to share the experience. When you hurt, they hurt. Your sad story becomes their sad story. "A Five is likely to cry when someone else cries," Spiegel notes, "even before knowing the cause of the tears. They have this wonderful way of empathizing. A very hypnotizable young woman I knew years ago would see a friend's dog being sick and immediately be nauseated herself. Empathy is a fine quality, of course, but it can be misplaced. A nurse, for example, who happens to be a Five had better train herself not to share the agony of her patients, otherwise she won't be around to help out.

"The incredible sensitivity of the Fives in picking up cues," as Spiegel puts it, is revealed in the case of a young Frenchwoman in her thirties who came to Dr. Barbara DeBetz in great distress because of her fear of being a lesbian. Even though she had led a completely "normal" sex life and had had only one homosexual experience (when she and another teenager practiced kissing in case they met any boys), several recent comments by men and advances by women had led her to accept the notion that she might be a lesbian. "I'm glad she came to see me," says DeBetz, "because I was able to identify her high hypnotizability and clarify the issue. She could so easily have let herself in for an endless round of psychotherapy that would seek to determine whether there was an important homosexual urge lurking in the background. Someone like this who is so responsive could have become confused and really started doubting her own feelings and judgment about her sexual nature."

Another important feature of the Highs is the telescoping of time. Their emphasis is mainly on the present. They are not much concerned about the past or future. They lack historical perspective as they make decisions (neglecting to remember an earlier bad experience, for example) and too often fail to anticipate the consequences of present actions. What counts is what is immediately before them, not what once happened or might happen.

"Paradoxically," Spiegel says, "the Fives, and only the Fives, are the people who can experience age regression so thoroughly that they relive the past in the present tense. When a Five regresses to his fourth birthday, it is experienced as a fourth birthday. Someone else may get a fragmentary experience but will remain aware of the present time and the fact that he is recalling an event of the past. The Fives have this amazing ability to recall layer upon layer of memory, but their tendency is to keep it all dormant and not apply the information to current decision making. And so the Five is prone to make the same mistake over and over again."

When motivated to learn something, the Fives are like sponges soaking up water. They take in information uncritically and may or may not appraise what they have absorbed later on. Insofar as there is such a thing as a photographic memory, it is the highly hypnotizable person who has it.

The possessor of a superb eidetic, or visual, memory has a great advantage over others, of course, but it is a mixed blessing. Spiegel tells of a young man—a straight-A student through high school and college—who found at Columbia's dental school that he could breeze through the examinations because he remembered every text and lecture. He could visualize whole pages of a book. "In the clinic, however, he proved to be awkward and clumsy when it came to translating this knowledge into finger movements. Typical of highly hypnotizable people, he had not integrated the information so that it mixed in with other knowledge. He knew the stuff but he didn't know what to do with it. He had to learn the material all over again, but this time thinking about it while taking it in."

Then there was the Five at medical school who became anxious and depressed after his anatomy professor singled him out for praise because of the perfect grade he had achieved on a difficult examination about the brachial plexus. "He got into an acute panic because he felt like a cheat. He knew he wasn't the best student in the class. By dumb luck he had looked at a diagram of the brachial plexus before the examination. He saw it so clearly in his mind that all he had to do, he said, was 'simply copy' the diagram."

The Fives, above all, have an outstanding capacity for concentration and dissociation. Even without formal hypnosis, they are able to step out of themselves, so to speak, just as the captain of an airliner can put the plane on automatic pilot while he attends to other things. Spiegel cites the artists and writers who tell of their paintings and novels coming into being while they look on as fascinated spectators. "I remember a painter who said, 'I kept admiring my hand. I was awed by what it was doing.' Another time, a novelist told me about becoming so intrigued by one of the characters in a book she was writing that she stayed up all night following this character around to see what he would do next. It is this kind of intense concentration that makes the creator able to be with his creation and alongside it at the same time—to relate to that concentration in a guided, disciplined, yet dissociated way. It is also the critical feature that characterizes the perceptual alteration common to all hypnosis: the observed motor phenomena are secondary to the perceptual shift."

The Fives are relatively comfortable with—or unaware of—logical incongruity. "They remind me of Tevye, the milkman in *Fiddler on the Roof*," Spiegel says. "In one of Sholem Aleichem's stories, Tevye is arbitrating between two friends who have taken opposite positions in an argument. He listens to the first man and says, 'You're right!' Then he listens to the second man and says, 'You're right!' When a third man protests that this is illogical because they both can't be right, Tevye says, 'You're right!'"

Hypnosis researchers speak of the phenomenon of "trance logic." It appears, for example, in the case of a hypnotized person accepting the assertion that the individual he sees sitting in a chair to his right is also sitting in the empty chair to his left. In short, he hallucinates a second figure. When asked how it is possible for someone to be in two places at once, he may well provide an inventive "logical" explanation. Even if he cannot explain it, he remains untroubled by the incongruity.

Trance logic appears outside the trance state as well, and it is particularly evident in the Fives. Their inclination is blithely to accept statements and viewpoints—as expressed, say, by a cult leader or an advocate of a conspiracy theory—that more skeptical people would reject as absurd. They would not be as likely as others, for example, to question the assertion of a Vietnam War army officer that a village had to be destroyed in order to save it.

The trance logic of the Fives does not show up so frequently or dramatically in less hypnotizable persons, Spiegel explains, because they do not swallow wholesale what they see or hear. "Because they are prone to assay critically each new life experience as it unfolds, the people who are not so trance-prone usually retain a judgmental distillate of the event rather than the entire detailed sequence and its effects. They focus more on derivation than on affiliation; hence past-time perspective remains intact."

In therapy, Spiegel observes, a Five can be extraordinarily accommodating as he or she puts great trust in the therapist, "but underneath this wonderful, malleable overlay is a narrow, hard, *fixed* core: a dynamism so fixed that it is subject to neither negotiation nor change." A certain role confusion and sense of inferiority may come from this mixture of chameleonlike changeability and hard-core dynamism. Even if a Five should perform so competently or creatively that he evokes praise from others, the dissociation from the performance is such that there is little recognition that "I" did it. "It" just happened. The author of a best-selling novel may feel embarrassed about his success because his characters came out of nowhere and made up the dialogue that he wrote down. The medical student who could "see" the anatomy diagram during an examination believed that he had done nothing himself and did not deserve top marks.

The characteristics that are so pronounced in the Fives provided a starting point for Spiegel when he decided to seek out the personality features of those at the other end of the spectrum of hypnotizability.

The opposite numbers of the Fours and Fives, whom he called the Highs, were the Zeros and Ones, otherwise known as the Lows. If the Highs could be described as heart people (who let feelings come before thought), then the Lows figured to be head people or brain people. And so Spiegel found them to be. He characterizes the Lows as more rational than emotional, more guarded than trusting, more controlled than impulsive. Their feet are on the ground.

"The Lows put tremendous emphasis on reason and understanding," he says. "They are extremely prone to planning for the future and employing their critical faculties to the utmost." The Lows are verbal types: good explainers who seek explanations. Whereas a High will go into hypnosis without first asking a lot of questions about it, the Low may well initiate such a discussion that the therapist must cut it short in order to get on with the job. Once cured of whatever has troubled him, a Low—in contrast to the indifference of a High—is likely to be interested in continuing in therapy in order to get to the roots of the problem. Spiegel learned years ago that the "why" therapy of psychoanalysis, as he calls it, is far more suitable to the Lows than to the Highs.

The impulse of the Lows to be in charge, to take control, not to give in to others except for well-calculated reasons, is often expressed in their zest for competition. "For many years," Spiegel relates, "I enjoyed the company of a very successful businessman whose idea of recreation was to go sailing in his forty-four-foot yawl. Because I often went along as the crew, he used to go around bragging that he had the only yacht on Long Island Sound with a staff psychiatrist. This man had an eye roll of one. He was definitely an Apollonian. We would be sailing along on a nice summer afternoon and he'd look at another boat and say, 'That son of a bitch doesn't know it, but we're racing him!' He couldn't understand sailing just for the sake of sailing. Because the Lows tend to orient themselves to external things, their inclination is to compete—to measure themselves against others. The Highs, on the other hand, are so absorbed in their own reactions and experiences as they perceive and deal with the world around them that it doesn't occur to them that they might be in competition with someone else."

As he pondered the contrasting personalities of the Highs and Lows, Spiegel realized that they reflected a basic human dichotomy that has found its most vivid expression in Greek mythology. Apollo was the god of light, order, reason, and moderation. Dionysus was the god of wine, excess, fancy, and fertility. Borrowing his terms from the Greeks, Nietzsche said in *The Birth of Tragedy* that "the continuous development of art is bound up with the *Apollonian* and *Dionysian* duality." He contrasted the "Apollonian art of sculpture" with the "nonplastic, Dionysian art of music."

In Nietzsche's philosophy, Apollonians represent critical-rational power as opposed to the creative-imaginative power of the Dionysians. On the one hand, there is the "measured restraint" and "freedom from the wilder emotions" of Apollo; on the other hand, the "barbaric" Dionysian impulses that lead to "complete self-forgetfulness." The Dionysian expresses a kind of drunken frenzy and "a desire to sink back into the original oneness of nature." Operating on his instincts, the Dionysian does not hesitate to gratify his urges. His antithesis, the Apollonian, rises above raw nature and basic passions. He brings form and discipline to art. Nietzsche was ever mindful of the need to reconcile Dionysian passion and Apollonian control.

It seemed to Spiegel that "Apollonian" and "Dionysian" would make suitable labels for the hypnotizable extremes: those who were either exceptionally inhibited or exceptionally uninhibited in their eye rolls and personalities. The Lows certainly manifested the "measured restraint" of the Apollonians described by Nietzsche. And when the Highs rolled their eyes out of sight and plunged into the trance state, they certainly displayed the "complete self-forgetfulness" of Nietzsche's Dionysians.

As a psychiatrist, Spiegel was particularly attracted to the Apollonian-Dionysian typology because the personality contrasts could be described without implying value judgments about mental health. He was aware that professionals as well as many laymen, when discussing the behavior or thinking styles of individuals, employed such shortcut descriptions as "manic," "obsessive," "hysterical," and "schizophrenic" even when they had no intention of implying a predominance of psychopathology. As umbrella labels for exaggerated personality types, Apollonian and Dionysian were neutral and nonclinical. There was no suggestion that one was better than the other. They were just different.

While refining his ideas about the personality features of the trance-state extremists, Spiegel came upon a telling reference to Apollonian and Dionysian qualities in a 1972 letter to the editor of *Science* magazine by Hungarian-born biologist Albert Szent-Györgyi, a winner of the Nobel Prize. Szent-Györgyi began by noting that various commentators had divided scientists into the classical and the romantic, the systematic and the intuitive, the Apollonian and the Dionysian. "These classifications," he continued, "reflect extremes of two different attitudes of the mind that can be found equally in art, painting, sculpture, music or dance. One could probably discover them in other alleys of life. In science the Apollonian tends to develop established lines to perfection, while the Dionysian rather relies on intuition and is more likely to open new, unexpected alleys for research."

Szent-Györgyi went on to say that support for scientific research mostly takes the form of grants, and that "the present methods of distributing grants unduly favor the

Apollonian. Applying for a grant begins with writing a project. The Apollonian clearly sees the future lines of his research and has no difficulty writing a clear project. Not so the Dionysian, who knows only the direction in which he wants to go out into the unknown; he has no idea what he is going to find there and how he is going to find it."

Spiegel also was intrigued by the use of the Apollonian-Dionysian model by *New York Times* critic Harold Schonberg in an article about two internationally known conductors, Herbert von Karajan and Georg Solti. "Two more dissimilar conductors cannot be imagined," he wrote. "In every aspect they represent opposite poles of music-making." Schonberg described Karajan as an objectivist, a literalist, an organizer, and a complete technician. "An air of ultra-efficiency permeates his work," and he has "tight emotional control." In contrast, Solti is dramatic, colorful, emotional, romantic. "He is much more a colorist than Karajan, and there is much more rhythmic drive to his conducting." Schonberg concluded that "Solti is Dionysus, Karajan is Apollo."

All typologies are suspect, of course. People are too complex to be lined up in neat, adjoining columns as introverts and extroverts, oral and anal types, inner-directed and outer-directed, Type A's and Type B's—or as Apollonians and Dionysians. Even so, a properly understood typology can be useful as a means of illuminating characteristics that are pronounced in some individuals but not in others. A few people are outstandingly (but not exclusively) Apollonian or Dionysian, but most of us are in the middle of the spectrum. We may lean toward one side or the other, but our overall style of thinking and behaving is a combination of the features of the extremes.

Spiegel was uncertain for some time about what to call

the mid-range majority: the Twos and Threes on the hyp-notizability scale. Then one day, in a conversation with Jacob Stern, a professor of classics at City College in New York, he described the tendency of his mid-range patients to vacillate between reason and emotion, between head and heart. Professor Stern suggested that he call them Odysseans after Homer's tragic hero Odysseus, a troubled wanderer of fluctuating moods who was capable of heroic behavior and profound despair.

This appealed to Spiegel because the people who oc-cupy the middle ground come into the world as complex beings—admixtures of Apollonian and Dionysian traits—who are fated to switch constantly back and forth be-tween the cerebral and emotional parts of their nature.

"For these individuals," the Spiegels write in *Trance and Treatment*, "the tension between reason and feeling is in some ways more troublesome than for Apollonians and Dionysians. Odysseans are less settled and more com-pelled to find a formula that Nietzsche described as the stuff of which tragedies are made. And yet these individ-uals are often productive, normal people who have the kinds of life crises that we have learned to identify as part of normal growth and development."

Herbert Spiegel himself, as a mid-range hypnotic sub-ject with a two-three eye roll, is described by his associ-ates as almost the epitome of the Odyssean personality. One colleague sees him as "part poet, part scientist." An-other says that "his open-mindedness is probably the salient feature. He's not fixed at any extreme." It is sig-nificant that he plays a leading role both in the Dionysian world of the intuitive therapists and the Apollonian world of the investigators of hypnotic phenomena.

11

PERSONALITY AND HYPNOTIZABILITY

In music one must think with the heart and
feel with the brain.

—GEORGE SZELL

In identifying the clusters of traits that characterize Dionysians, Apollonians, and Odysseans, Spiegel has drawn on his clinical experience, Hypnotic Induction Profiles of thousands of patients, independent diagnoses and psychological testing of many of the same individuals, answers to questionnaires, and a survey of the literature on hypnotizability, neurophysiology, and psychopathology. The result is his "cluster hypothesis," or a series of generalizations about personality features that are linked to trance capacity.

Something new, then, has been added to the world's knowledge of hypnosis: personality as a predictor of hypnotizability.

Hypnosis experts have always sensed that certain human traits correspond with trance capacity, but there has been little agreement on what they are. In recent decades, a number of laboratory researchers have isolated a few features that seem to be special to extremely trance-prone individuals. As a clinician whose research data is a by-product of his work with patients, Spiegel has gone further than anyone in identifying sets of specific characteristics common to those who range in trance capacity from low to medium to high.

His chief aim in this work has been to provide guidelines that a therapist can use to tune in to a patient's individual style of concentrating, processing information, and interacting with other people. A good clinician wants to know how to reach a patient, how to speak his language, how to get him to mobilize his own resources for healing. Appreciation of a person's particular set of traits is bound to help.

Spiegel devised a brief questionnaire—a "personality inventory"—for a therapist to use, if he or she wishes, before administering the Profile to a new patient. The therapist employs an accompanying scoring sheet to circle the letter A, O, or D (for Apollonian, Odyssean, or Dionysian) according to the answer to each of the questions. It is hardly a "scientific" survey, but it has proven to be effective in pointing out a predominance of Apollonian or Dionysian features, or an Odyssean mixture of traits. "It gives you a feeling about where you're going," Spiegel says, "and it has value for breaking the ice with the patient and getting across the idea of alternatives. Most people try to give honest answers. It's a useful thing to know if there is a discrepancy or a harmonious relationship between the responses and the Profile. If a Four gives you Apollonian answers—or if a One responds like a Dionysian—it may be that he has been taught or brought up to behave in a way that is not really natural to him. The eye roll and the other physical reactions of the Profile will reveal who he really is."

These are the questions:

1. As you concentrate on watching a movie or a play, do you get so absorbed in what is going on that you lose awareness of where you are?

If so, do you ever get so absorbed that when the curtain comes down you are surprised to realize you are sitting in a theater?

2. In general, as you perceive time, do you focus more of your attention upon the past, present, or future—or all three equally?

3. The French philosopher Pascal once said, "The heart has a mind which the brain does not understand." He said there are two kinds of mind: the heart-mind and the brain-mind. As you know yourself, which of these two minds do you give priority to?

4. As you relate to another person, do you prefer to control the interaction or do you prefer to let the other person take over if he or she wishes?

5. In your proneness or tendency to trust other people, where would you place yourself on a scale of average, above, or below?

6. As you are learning something new, do you tend to judge it critically at the time you are learning it, or do you accept it and perhaps judge it critically at a later time?

7. As you sense your responsibility for what you do, where do you place yourself on a scale of average, above, or below?

8. If you are learning something new and you know in advance that it is of such a nature that you can learn it clearly, safely, and equally well by either seeing it or touching it, which would you prefer—to see it or to touch it?

9. When you come up with a new idea, there are two parts to it: One is to dream it up, and the other is to

figure out how to do it. Of these two parts, which gives you a greater sense of fulfillment?

10. As you come up with or work out a new idea, is it necessary to write notes or do you feel your way through without writing?

"It is remarkable," Spiegel says, "how often an Apollonian or a Dionysian will hear these questions, answer right away, and then say something like, 'In such a short time you know me so well.' This is not true, of course; their assumption is that there is only one answer to each question. They think that their way is the only way of perceiving the world."

The Apollonian, for example, upon hearing the first question, about spatial awareness, cannot imagine losing himself so completely in a movie or a play that he is unaware of his surroundings. "This doesn't mean that he cannot concentrate," Spiegel explains. "Hypnotizability is a measure of the balance between focal attention and peripheral awareness. In the trance state, there is an emphasis on focal attention with a reduction of peripheral awareness. The Apollonian will typically never lose total peripheral awareness even though he may lose some. Even when he is focusing to the best of his ability he still knows where he is. The Dionysian, of course, answers the question with a yes, and when you go on to ask about being surprised to find yourself sitting in a theater, the Dionysian will smile as he says yes because it is all so familiar and because he likes that spaced-out feeling. If you ask the same thing of an Apollonian, he doesn't know what you're talking about."

In answer to the second question, on time perception, the Apollonian will say that he focuses much more of his attention on the past and future than on the present.

"Many Apollonians are so busy analyzing where they've been and where they're going," Spiegel comments, "that they forget to live in the present tense. In contrast, the Dionysians feel that everything is now."

The next six questions are designed to identify the way an individual perceives and deals with the world. Spiegel observes that "we all live by a cloud of fears, biases, prejudices, stories we hear, things we see, bits of hard knowledge we acquire, and so on." He calls this "a myth-belief constellation—a mixture of private assumptions about the world related to intrapsychic development, family beliefs, and cultural myths." It amounts to a personal premise system—consciously realized only in part—that Spiegel describes as a "metaphor mix." He agrees with Ortega y Gasset's observation that "the metaphor is probably the most fertile power that man possesses" and says that highly hypnotizable people "are the most prone to shift the components of this metaphor mix to reach new treatment goals." He seeks to know, through these questions, how an individual, as he goes through life, puts together the premises that he lives by. For the Dionysian, the emphasis is on gut feelings. For the Apollonian, reason is more valued than feeling. The Odyssean relates to others and acquires new information by a more even combination of emotional commitment and cognitive judgment.

In answer to question 3, then, Dionysians see themselves as operating mainly with a heart-mind while Apollonians consider themselves to be brain-minded.

On the matter of control, the Apollonian will admit that he has a strong preference for being in charge. The Dionysian will say that he does not mind someone else taking control. Half-jokingly, Spiegel tells his students that "two Apollonians going for a drive in the same car will argue about which one is going to do the driving. If you have an Apollonian and a Dionysian, the Apollonian will drive even if the Dionysian owns the car. And if you have two Dionysians, they'll both sit in the back seat."

As for trust, the Apollonian will admit his caution about trusting other people while the Dionysian will rate himself as above average in his tendency to trust others. "The Apollonian," says Spiegel, "wants to have more information that will answer his question, 'Do you deserve my trust?' The Dionysian simply starts with the premise, 'Why shouldn't I trust you?' "

On the matter of critical appraisal and learning style, the Apollonian makes an immediate judgment while learning something. The Dionysian accepts the information and judges it later, if at all. Spiegel observes that Apollonians, when dealing with a barrage of new information (e.g., hearing a lecture or cramming for an examination), are so busy appraising the data that they do not take it all in. The spongelike Dionysians just accept it all without using the filter of judgment. Apollonians may not have the Dionysian knack for recalling data but they are much better at integrating new information with old information for sound decision making.

"The Dionysian," Spiegel explains, "affiliates with the information he acquires but he doesn't connect it as well to what he already knows. So it's like a Chinese meal: It doesn't stick to the ribs. However, this is not the case in his professional life. In those areas where he functions as an expert, where he is expected to make sound judgments, the Dionysian can be as discerning as an Apollonian. It is only in the peripheral areas that he is more accepting.

"For example, there is a doctor I know here in New York who has an eye roll of four. He happens to be a world authority in his specialty. He is also an expert on puts and calls in the stock market. In fact, he is so successful in the market that he can afford to finance his own medical research. So in these two areas he is sharp and critical. Nobody can put anything over on him. But outside of these areas he is like putty in the hands of a persuasive person. When he takes a day off and walks around the city, looking into stores, he ends up buying television sets, refrigerators, furniture, and other stuff that he doesn't need. One of his wife's jobs is to send back the things he buys because he can't say no to salesmen."

On the question of responsibility, Spiegel allows that many people would not wish to admit to being less than responsible. Still, he finds that Apollonians, in contrast to their opposite numbers, take a particular pride in being responsible. "Dionysians, who do not seek a reputation for being a Rock of Gibraltar, are more inclined to intense, short-term involvements rather than long-run commitments. Moreover, they tend to look to others to furnish guidelines for appropriate conduct rather than cling to their own certainties." In working with patients who wish to give up smoking, Spiegel has found that Dionysians will often agree with alacrity to a stop-smoking procedure and then fail to follow through. In contrast, Apollonians will be cautious about making a commitment but more likely to see it through.

As for question 8 about mode of contact (the last of the questions dealing with the myth-belief constellation), the Apollonian prefers to see or visualize the thing he is learning while the Dionysian's preference is to touch it. In a museum, the first will be content to study a work of sculpture at a distance while the second may feel an irresistible urge to put his hands on it.

Questions 9 and 10 of Spiegel's personality inventory are concerned with differing styles of behavioral processing or implementing ideas. In general, Dionysians find greater fulfillment in dreaming up an idea; Apollonians achieve satisfaction in figuring out how to carry out an idea. The Dionysian architect whose genius lies in creating imaginative structures may be uninterested in the actual business of construction. He will happily leave such things to his Apollonian colleagues.

As might be expected, Apollonians are great note takers and list makers. They like to put their ideas into writing. The Dionysian feels his way through without having to write things down. Spiegel recalls one Apollonian patient who came to him because of his smoking habit. "After I told him the instructions that he could give himself when using self-hypnosis, he asked if I had them in writing. I said I didn't but I could let him have a recording of the instructions. That would be fine, he said. Then he asked me if it would be okay if he transcribed the record."

Although there are some people who respond to the personality questions in an all-Apollonian or all-Dionysian fashion, most people reveal in their answers a more balanced mixture of traits—a sign of mid-range hypnotizability and an overall Odyssean personality. Odyssean answers tend to be ambiguous. When asked whether they like to control an interaction or let someone else take over, they may say that it depends on the situation. They trust people, but only moderately; they see themselves as moderately responsible; they find fulfillment both in developing and implementing new ideas; they have no special preference for tactile or visual learning, or for oral or visual language; and so it goes.

Because Odysseans are a blend of opposites, they usually succeed in functioning comfortably in settings that put a premium on Apollonian or Dionysian qualities. It is a different story for the Apollonian who is expected to behave as a Dionysian or for the Dionysian trying to survive in an Apollonian atmosphere.

Dr. DeBetz remembers meeting a woman who had grown up in a small town in Sicily before coming to the United States to practice medicine. "She had a low eye roll and Apollonian traits and yet she came from a Dionysian culture. While in Italy she had made an effort to behave as a Dionysian but she always had a feeling of being displaced. She told me that she felt a great sense of relief in America because for the first time she didn't have to pretend to be the romantic, heart-oriented person that Italians are supposed to be. Now she could be a practical-minded Apollonian without feeling uncomfortable about it. Her husband said that in Italy she was 'like a fish out of water.' "

DeBetz added: "I know what that fish-out-of-water feeling is like. I'm on the high side of the hypnotizability scale but I come from Germany, an Apollonian culture. In medical school I had the advantage of a Dionysian's memory but I had to learn to discipline myself and fit into the structure. So both of us, as different types coming from very different cultures, came to the United States, where we could be ourselves because there are no specific expectations about what a person should be like."

Some people with strong Apollonian or Dionysian qualities achieve a balance in their lives through association with their opposite numbers. Spiegel was drawn to a *New York Times Magazine* article on Dr. Rosalyn Yalow, a winner of the 1977 Nobel Prize in medicine, because of its description of her twenty-two-year partnership in medical research with the late Dr. Solomon Berson. The man responsible for bringing the two together, Dr. Bernard Straus, was quoted as saying that the collaboration was a "combination of poetry and pottery. He provided the biological brilliance, and she the mathematical muscle. Berson was something of a romantic. Dr. Yalow was keen and scientific, certainly a steadying influence."

Discussions of personality in these terms inevitably inspire speculation about the marriage, say, of two Dionysians or two Apollonians. Is a hypnotic High more likely to find happiness with a Low or a Mid-range or another High? Are people better off marrying their likes or their opposites? Do Odysseans achieve harmony when they marry each other or do their vacillating natures lead to conflict?

Spiegel knows there are no easy answers and makes no recommendations. Even so, the physicians who attend his Columbia course will often seize on this subject for their coffee-break discussions. One day, a young physician from Ohio spoke of his Apollonian characteristics, while his Dionysian wife stood at his side, nodding agreement. "I'm a Gordon Liddy type," he asserted. "I'd go through that wall over there if I had to. I spend a hundred percent of my time controlling. I worry about it, though. I don't want to be as vulnerable as a Five but I realize that you just can't always control people. If I really want to do something and my wife doesn't, she's the one who will give in. Just the same, we get along fine. In fact, it's a good thing we're both not Dionysian. She can't structure herself. If we've got to be somewhere at six o'clock, she's still doing the dishes at ten minutes to six. With her, everything is right now. With me, the present is not something I worry about. I've got that under control and I'm thinking about what to do next. Somebody's got to make the decisions."

The doctor said that he would like to be more Dionysian than he is—though not too much; he clearly took pride in his Apollonian qualities. The doctor's wife, though content with being a Dionysian, said it would be nice to be a little more Apollonian.

But can people change? To a limited extent, Spiegel says, if they really wish to do so. "Centering" is one kind of therapy for Highs and Lows with psychological problems: encouraging them to shift toward the Odyssean middle by putting greater emphasis on neglected qualities of mind. The Dionysian can make greater use of his critical skills; the Apollonian can become more sensitive to feelings.

Charles Darwin had something to say on the matter a century ago: "If I had my life to live over again, I would have made a rule to read some poetry and listen to some music at least once a week; for perhaps the parts of my brain now atrophied would have thus been kept active through use. The loss of these tastes is a loss of happiness, and may possibly be injurious to the intellect, and more probably to the moral character, by enfeebling the emotional part of our nature."

12

NO SMOKING

To acquire a new habit is easy, because one
main function of the nervous system is to act
out as a habit-forming machine; to break out
of a habit is an almost heroic feat of mind or
character.

—ARTHUR KOESTLER,
*The Art of
Creation*

A well-dressed lady from the South appeared in Dr. Spiegel's office one day and told him, "You have been given to
me as my birthday present."

She explained that she was Catherine Meacham, the
fashion editor of the Memphis *Press-Scimitar*, and she
was in New York because her daughter and son-in-law
were concerned about her cigarette habit. As a gift, they
had arranged this appointment to see if hypnosis could be
the means to get her to give up smoking.

When Spiegel asked her to do an eye roll, her eyes did
not move. When he led her through the Profile test, she
did not go into trance. She was an Intact Zero. "How did I
do?" she asked. "I can't hypnotize you," he said. Her
sense of relief was obvious. She had come with the belief
that going into trance implied weakness of mind or want
of intelligence. At the same time, she was disappointed
because of the expectations of her daughter and son-in-
law and the expense and trouble they had gone to. Then
Spiegel asked her if she would like to learn the strategy

for mastering the smoking habit, saying, "You can use it even if you're not hypnotizable." She said she was eager to hear it.

For the next half hour, Spiegel talked to Mrs. Meacham about herself as an individual who is much more than a person who smokes cigarettes, and about her relationship to her body and her responsibilities to her body. As she wrote later on in her newspaper, "He asked me questions, such as, 'Wouldn't I take care of a child if it were left on my doorstep? Why wouldn't I take care of my own person!' It went on and on! I found it very silly, a little tiresome. And then he ushered me out. I remember I kept saying how sorry I was he could not hypnotize me; what would I tell my children; would it be all right if I pretended to be cured."

She told her daughter and son-in-law of her disappointment. "I apologized profusely. I thanked them for thinking of such a wonderful present and told them how sorry I was that it had not worked."

Later that night, after dining at a restaurant, "I realized I had not smoked one cigarette. Usually at a dinner I would have smoked at least four." The next day, when she attended a fashion showing, "I did not even think about smoking, though all day long I was surrounded by women puffing away, their smoke blowing in my face, their cigarettes dangling almost under my nose."

She was so amazed and perplexed by this experience that she wrote a two-thousand-word article about it when she returned to Memphis.

"For 30 years," she began, "I have smoked cigarettes, the first 15 years a pack a day and the last 15 two or three packs a day. In that period I estimate I smoked nearly 25,000 packages. I do not smoke any more. I stopped at 5 P.M. Friday, June 20, when I visited a New York doctor and he hypnotized me. Now, when I put a cigarette to my lips, there is no feeling. When I try to puff, I cannot inhale. The desire is sometimes there but no longer amenable to smoke."

(A decade later, when contacted by the author, she said she had never resumed smoking, "and a good thing too because I surely would have had emphysema.")

Although Mrs. Meacham clearly was delighted to be a sudden nonsmoker, she ended her article by saying, "I keep wondering why that doctor tricked me. Why did he tell me he could not hypnotize me? How did he do it?"

Says Spiegel: "I didn't do it; she did it. I didn't hypnotize her, because she couldn't be hypnotized. But I did tell her that you don't have to be hypnotizable to get a therapeutic effect if you have enough motivation. She was deeply motivated by the love that her daughter and her son-in-law were expressing to her by arranging for this experience. She adopted a whole new outlook about her body, apparently without realizing it. She was sure that I had somehow tricked her into hypnosis. But remember that there are unconscious as well as conscious processes at work all the time. Alfred North Whitehead once said, 'Reason is the horse we ride after we have decided which direction we want to go.' "

For most of the smokers who come to Spiegel (and to other clinicians who have adopted his approach), hypnosis plays a key role in imbedding a new point of view in the mind and reinforcing it later on; but what happened to Mrs. Meacham might be called hypnosis without hypnosis. Her wish to succeed was so great that she was able to shift into a new, smokeless life-style even without the extra thrust of the trance state. Spiegel's role was pretty much that of a sparkplug for an engine that was primed to go. In a different but related instance, a researcher for a national magazine interviewed him for an article about stress. Her curiosity about his innovative approach to the smoking habit was aroused. She went home with copies of articles in professional journals about his respect-your-body strategy. Whereupon she quit smoking.

Every lay and professional therapist, whether geared to hypnosis or not, can, of course, produce success stories about his or her smoking-control method. Many outlandish claims are made, even though the difficulty of getting "hard-core" smokers to stop smoking is well known. Published reports of results tend to be highly anecdotal. Little is said about failures, in part because few therapists make any attempt to do long-range follow-up studies. In this regard, Spiegel is extraordinary. He has made extensive and expensive efforts to keep in touch with patients, record short-term and long-term results, and publish his findings for professional appraisal. As various commentators have noticed, he has been almost too conservative in reporting the percentage of successful treatments.

Most smokers who quit smoking, of course, do so on their own. Many smokers do not wish to give up tobacco and make no effort to stop even if they understand the risks. The hard-core smokers are those who want to stop, who have tried to stop, but who cannot stop. They frustrate the family doctors who try to help them. So great is the frustration, wrote Spiegel years ago, that "many physicians stop telling their patients about the dangers of smoking. The usual suggestion to 'cut down' conveys an ill-disguised helplessness. Patients perceive this suggestion as the mildest of rebukes and one that merely telegraphs the message: 'I am resigned to the reality that you are unable to stop smoking.' "

Such patients are the ones that Spiegel sees. One fifty-seven-year-old man, a three-packs-a-day smoker, said he had been smoking since he was ten years old. Yet the treatment Spiegel offers is provided in just one forty-five-minute encounter instead of the customary multiple sessions of stop-smoking therapy. Despite its brevity, his method produces results that are comparable to and often superior to more conventional and time-consuming procedures described in the professional literature.

"There is a big difference in response," Spiegel says, "between patients with Intact profiles who can fully express their trance potential and the Nonintact people who cannot. We have follow-up data on more than a thousand cases. For the Intact patients, whether low, mid-range, or high in trance capacity, the short-term results are very impressive. Two thirds of them stop smoking after the one visit. But there is a lot of backsliding in the first three months. By six months to a year later, when stabilization of the permanent response emerges, we find that 31 to 32 percent are successful. So the bottom line is that one out of three of the Intact patients becomes a nonsmoker for the long run. Those with Soft profiles, who can only partially express their trance potential, succeed at about an 18 percent rate. As for the Decrement patients who have the biological equipment for hypnosis but cannot use it, only 7 percent stop smoking permanently with this approach.

"The sad truth is that not all people are able to change—even a habit as destructive as this. The figures show, for example, that childless adults who are divorced or widowed are notoriously unsuccessful in dealing with smoking. Unlike parents who realize that they are setting a bad example for their children, or who have been implored by their children to stop smoking, these people don't come in with the same motivation and commitment.

"The single treatment is a practical way of salvaging

those who can respond, and, because it is only one session, the therapist's time is not saturated with an accumulation of nonresponders."

One of Spiegel's "failures" was a world-famous journalist and author in his seventies who was suffering from severe bronchitis and coronary heart disease. Despite his terrible cough and worsening condition, he would not stop smoking. His physician, an old friend, threatened to have nothing further to do with him unless he agreed to see Dr. Spiegel and give hypnosis a try.

When the writer arrived at Spiegel's office, his opening words were, "How do you do, doctor? I'm not glad to meet you." In an amiable but firm manner, he made it clear that he had lived a long and rewarding life, he had made arrangements for the care of his family, and he had no intention of giving up cigarettes.

"As long as you're here," Spiegel said, "would you like to hear what the strategy is?" "Of course," replied the old reporter. "Would you mind if I take notes?" This was a clue that he was probably an Apollonian—as he proved to be. His eye roll was that of a One. When Spiegel began to speak about respecting and protecting one's body, the author dropped his note pad and exclaimed, "Don't give me that Albert Schweitzer crap! Schweitzer was the biggest boob I ever met in my life!" Spiegel said he was not talking about "reverence for life" but about the simple fact that "you can't live without your body." To which the patient replied that he had a right to decide how long he wanted to live. "But don't you have a few more books in you?" Spiegel asked. "That may be," he was told, "but I can assure you, doctor, that the world will get along just as well without them." Six months later the writer was dead.

Spiegel was himself a smoker until the early 1960s

when the evidence about the harmful effects of cigarette smoking began to accumulate. This personal turn of events coincided with his shift away from long-term analysis to briefer forms of psychotherapy and his growing interest in preventive medicine. Patients came to him with all kinds of problems, and very often he felt that the best thing he could do for them was to help them overcome a health-destroying, life-shortening habit. Later on, when he had developed his technique for smothering the smoking urge with positive, life-enhancing urges, he felt even more strongly about devoting a lot more of his clinical time to this side of medicine—a side that most psychiatrists choose to ignore or think is unworthy of their special skills. Most satisfying of all was the evidence of psychological dividends produced by the mastery of a bad habit. "If I can do this," the typical patient came to believe, "then I can do other things. I can take charge of my life. I can be a different me."

The ripple effect was demonstrated by a patient who came to Spiegel in the first place not to stop smoking but to "sharpen my concentration." She was a legal secretary who was ambitious to be a free-lance court reporter. She faced a tough examination and wanted to bring all her resources to bear on the questions. Profiling as a highly motivated Two, she was taught the screen technique: imagining a personal movie screen, projecting the course material onto it, and giving the data the undivided attention that the trance state makes possible. She passed the exams handsomely.

"What really amazed me about this," she says, "was that I practically stopped smoking. I was down to four cigarettes a day instead of two packs a day and yet I hadn't gone to see Dr. Spiegel about my smoking habit. He did say, however, when I asked him if it would be okay if I smoked while we talked, that it bothered him to see people committing suicide. Others had told me that smoking was bad for me but this time it really must have sunk in."

Unfortunately, the virtual conquest of her smoking habit was accompanied by a steady increase in her weight. She called Spiegel about it, and he agreed to see her for a second session. It was his opinion that the weight increase amounted to "unconscious sabotage" to give herself a reason to start smoking again. "She was telling herself, 'I won't smoke, and thus was fighting it. Because of the fighting, she was eating more. I decided to give her the restructuring strategy. We discussed protecting the body from both smoking and overeating, and we talked about thin-eating and fat-eating. Since this was riding on the momentum of the change in her that had already taken place, I wasn't surprised that it worked."

She began to lose weight and stopped smoking completely. She remembers going to her car after that second session and experiencing a wild desire to throw away the cigarettes in her pocketbook. She did throw them out. "Then I saw a man going to his car, smoking, and I thought to myself, 'He's a smoker, but I'm different.' I didn't envy him." Later on, when she noticed her weight going down, "my first reaction was a great sense of accomplishment. To lose weight and not smoke at the same time seemed incredible. I had this wonderful feeling of not being able to wait to see what I would do next."

Some years before developing the unusual strategy that he describes as "restructuring," Spiegel took steps to reduce the treatment time involved in smoking control. It has been customary for smokers who sign up for therapy—whether with a private practitioner or an organization like Smokenders that operates group-therapy programs—to spend a number of days or weeks, at no small expense, reinforcing their commitment to a tobacco-less life.

"In the days when I was using an aversion method for smoking," Spiegel recalls, "I was still influenced by my analytic training. I figured you keep trying and trying until you get some result. But I had one man who was still smoking after five sessions and when he was due to appear in my office for the sixth time I had a fantasy about a hole in the floor that I could drop through—that's how much I didn't want to see him. When he appeared, I leveled with him. I said I would see him one more time and no more. This would be our final session no matter what happened. He stopped smoking as soon as he realized that there was a limit to the treatment. I realized that if a patient thought that ten visits to the doctor were necessary, for smoking or anything else, then it would take ten visits. If he knew the treatment would be limited to one visit, then, if he was going to stop at all, one visit would be enough."

The obvious benefit of single-session therapy, with the patient carrying on the treatment with self-hypnosis, was that many more patients could be seen in the time that normally was taken with one patient. Compressing the time involved made it all the more imperative that the right kind of message be conveyed to the smoker. In common with other practitioners who used hypnosis to give added leverage to the therapy, Spiegel's strategy at the time put greater emphasis on the things the patient should be *against*, not on what he should be *for*. The patient, after learning that he should be against smoking because of the harm it does, would be conditioned to resist the smoking urge and view smoking as an unpleasant experience. This was sometimes an effective method, but Spiegel, especially after telephoning a number of patients to check on the long-term results, felt it was not good enough. He also sensed that there should be more accent on the positive instead of the negative.

"There was one man who taught me a good lesson," he says. "He was a big Italian with the build of a football player. He was sure I could help him because I was connected with the hospital, Columbia Presbyterian, that his father's contracting company had built. He desperately wanted to give up smoking because it was ruining the arteries in his legs so badly that when he walked two blocks the pain would force him to stop and rest.

"This was before I cut down on multiple sessions and before I developed the Profile, but almost surely he was a One or a Two—definitely on the low side. After several appointments he was still smoking, and I had to tell him that we were getting nowhere. He told me it was just as well because he was going on vacation. When I found out that he was heading for Arizona I suggested that he go see Milton Erickson. I told him that Erickson was a great doctor, a famous therapist, who got wonderful results with hypnosis.

"I learned later that when he appeared in Erickson's office with three packs of cigarettes in his pockets he was surprised to see Erickson, who had been ill and in pain for many years, sitting in a wheelchair. After that first visit, he stopped smoking. He was still not smoking when he returned to Erickson for two more sessions. When he came back to New York he thanked me profusely for sending him to the great Arizona doctor. His smoking days were over.

"The following year, when Erickson came to New York to lecture at my course, I thought I would surprise him by bringing in this patient and let Erickson tell the audience how he had succeeded where I had failed. But first I asked the patient to tell us what happened down there in Arizona. He said, 'You mean you want me to tell the truth about what happened?' I said, 'Sure, tell us the truth.' So he said, "Well, I went to Doc Spiegel six or seven times and he couldn't do anything for me but when he sent me to Doc Erickson I stopped smoking after just one session.'

"I asked him if there was any difference in the hypnosis. He said it was the same. 'Then why,' I asked, 'did you stop smoking with Dr. Erickson and not with me?'

" 'All right,' he said, 'I'll tell you the truth,' and when he did there were tears in his eyes. 'When I went all the way to Arizona and saw this nice, gray-haired man sitting in a wheelchair with crippled legs, I could only think that here's this old man whose legs are useless trying to help a big bull of a guy like me save his legs. That really got me! I realized that I wasn't respecting my body.'

"Well, that's where the phrase comes from. He learned to respect his body, and to stop smoking, by just the emotional experience of seeing this crippled man in a wheelchair going to all the trouble of trying to help him.

"After this I started to shift my whole point of view about how to help people stop smoking. It took a while to develop the concept of respecting your body so that people could really understand and absorb it. There had to be a setup first: pointing out that smoking is poison to your body and you need your body to live. After that is understood, the commitment is: To the extent you want to live, you owe your body this respect.

"At about the time that I noticed it was working with patients, David, who was studying philosophy at Yale, was home on vacation. I told him about this great discovery: Instead of fighting the symptom you put it in a positive way by affirming your commitment to your body. David said to me, 'Gee, Dad, I don't want to hurt your feelings, but Hegel wrote about that a long time ago.'

"He was speaking, of course, about Hegel's way of setting up a dialectic when you have a dilemma and looking for the affirmation that comes out of the dialectic. In the case of someone who wants to quit smoking yet likes to smoke, the challenge is to formulate the problem in such a way that the resolution is an affirmation experience instead of a fight. You don't fight the urge to smoke. The urge is there but there is also a desire not to smoke, perhaps because you have taken the statistics on lung cancer to heart or because your children have been pleading with you to quit."

The strategic mistake for a therapist talking to a patient, or a patient talking to himself, Spiegel believes, is to say, Don't smoke! "Unless you're a masochist, that doesn't work. If you feel that not smoking is punishment and you enjoy being punished, then you might stop smoking. If not, the odds are that the more you say, Don't smoke!, the more you want to smoke, and you probably will."

A popular aversive technique used by professional and lay practitioners who employ hypnosis is the posthypnotic suggestion that cigarettes smell and taste like horse manure, or something equally offensive. It is an approach that can work for some people, at least for a time. It can even work too well. One psychiatrist who used this approach received a frantic telephone call from the patient some hours later. "My house smells awful," the man complained. "Why?" the doctor asked. "Are you still smoking?" Said the patient, "No, but my wife is." The psychiatrist was obliged to modify the suggestion so that the only foul smells would be those coming from cigarettes that the patient personally smoked.

The trouble with such a method, Spiegel feels, is that it does not instill a genuine conviction about the value of not smoking and the virtue of taking care of one's body. The patient has been conned into believing that tobacco is as foul as manure, but it really isn't true, as part of his mind knows, and the passage of time or a counterinfluence can make smoking pleasurable once again. Or else, because the patient has been denied one kind of gratification, he may quickly turn to another or otherwise give expression to his frustration. He probably has heard that a display of withdrawal symptoms is expected of the smoker who makes the ultimate sacrifice. He may start eating everything in sight and be bad-tempered with family and friends—so much so that everyone will implore him to start smoking again.

A far better approach, Spiegel has found, is to create an affirmation experience. "That's good primary strategy for many things, whether you use hypnosis or not. But with hypnosis you get extra impact."

Spiegel's stance with a smoking patient is one of "respectful impatience," as if saying that if you really want to give up cigarettes, let's get on with it and get it done. The time is now! There is going to be one session and then you are on your own. Only a brief clinical history is taken: how many years of smoking, average number of cigarettes, physical symptoms, how many others in the household smoke, and so on. The HIP and cluster survey are used to assess trance capacity and personality. If the patient is an Apollonian, Spiegel will put things more in terms of puzzle solving. With a Dionysian, there is greater emphasis on the emotional appeal of protecting the body's innocence. The presentation to Odysseans varies.

As the patient emerges from the trance experience at the completion of the Profile test, Spiegel takes the opportunity to point out that hypnosis is not sleep but a method of concentration that "enables you to be optimally receptive to your own thoughts. The strategy that you use in this receptive atmosphere is what we take up next."

He shows the patient how to put himself into trance because he will be expected to do so periodically to reinforce his new commitment. Now that the patient is again hypnotized, Spiegel says: "In this state of meditation, you concentrate on the feeling of floating and, at the same time, concentrate on these three critical points.

"The first point is: For your body, smoking is a poison. You are composed of a number of components, the most important of which is your body. Smoking is not so much a poison for you as it is for your body specifically.

"The second point is: You cannot live without your body. Your body is a precious physical plant through which you experience life.

"The third point is: To the extent that you want to live, you owe your body respect and protection. This is your way of acknowledging the fragile, precious nature of your body, and at the same time, your way of seeing yourself as your body's keeper. You are, in truth, your body's keeper. When you make this commitment to respect your body, you have within you the power to have smoked your last cigarette.

"Notice how this strategy puts the emphasis on what you are for, rather than what you are against. It is true that smoking is a poison and you are against it, but the emphasis is upon the commitment to respect your body. As a consequence of your commitment, it becomes natural for you to protect your body against the poison of further smoking.

"Observe that when you make this commitment to respect your body, you incorporate with it a view toward eating and drinking that reflects your respect for your body. As a result, each eating and drinking experience in itself creates an exercise in disciplined concern for your body. You can, if you wish, use this same exercise to maintain your ideal weight while protecting your body against the poison of further smoking."

Spiegel goes on to propose that the patient do this self-hypnosis as often as ten times a day, at least in the beginning, preferably every one or two hours. He does not say how long the patient should continue the self-hypnotic reinforcements. The need for them fades away with the smoking urge but the ex-smoker may well decide to carry on his occasional moments of relaxation and introspection.

Spiegel tells the patient that the exercise, which takes about a minute at first but only twenty seconds with practice, is simply a matter of going into trance, letting one arm float to an upright position as a signal for meditation, and then concentrating on the three critical points: "For my body, smoking is a poison. I need my body to live. I owe my body this respect and protection." After reflecting on "what this means to you in a private sense," the final step is to emerge from the state of concentration while retaining a general feeling of floating.

Because the patient has been carrying out these directions as they are given, he now is out of hypnosis but he continues to listen attentively. "This floating sensation," Spiegel says, "signals your mind to turn inward and pay attention to your own thoughts—like private meditation. Ballet dancers and athletes float all the time. That is why they concentrate and coordinate their movements so well. When they do not float they are uptight and they do not do as well."

He explains that the reason for doing the exercise regularly ("Your body is entitled to twenty seconds every one or two hours") is to reimprint the three points, like reinforcing a program in a computer. "If I had my way," he adds, "I would ask you to spend the next week living in a tobacco shop to emphasize the point that the issue is not the presence of tobacco but rather your private commitment to your body even in the presence of tobacco. Smokers can stop smoking if you lock them in a room and don't give them tobacco, but that in no way internalizes the change. You know that you are internalizing the change when in the presence of tobacco you decide to give priority to your body."

When speaking to Apollonian smokers, Spiegel challenges them to solve a geometric puzzle: connecting nine dots arranged in three parallel rows by using four connected straight lines, all without lifting the pencil from the paper.

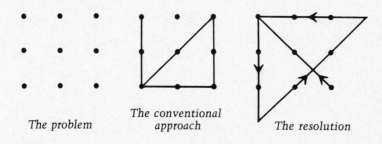

The problem   The conventional approach   The resolution

This makes the point that the smoking problem should be approached from the outside and not in conventional terms of smoking or not smoking. It should be viewed in terms of taking responsibility for one's body. In this way, the smoking habit is controlled indirectly. It falls by the wayside as attention is paid to more important matters.

For Dionysians and most Odysseans, Spiegel seeks a more emotional response: "Look at yourself in this double sense: There is you and your body. You are your body's keeper, and your body is your physical plant. There is something precious and helpless about your body. It is just like with a baby. When you put poison into your body it can do nothing but accept it and make the best of it. But when you realize that you are the one putting the poison there, you have some questions to ask yourself. Which side are you on? Are you for your body or are you not? Are you for living or are you not? If you are not for living, keep on smoking. But if the idea of living is still enticing, then you have a built-in obligation to give your body the respect that it deserves."

(A few years ago in Florida, when Spiegel spent most of a week teaching hypnosis to a gathering of doctors, a physician who said he wished to quit the habit volunteered to take part in a demonstration of smoking control. He was a prime hypnotic subject—an Intact Four. He learned the strategy as described here. And yet when he was asked some days later to appear on the platform for a follow-up discussion, he said he was still smoking. Spiegel invited the audience to join him in analyzing this case. One doctor asked the smoker whether he had any fear of dying. "None at all," the man said. He was very religious; he believed strongly in the hereafter; he did not fear death from cancer or anything else. Spiegel now realized that he would have to adjust his approach. He knew the physician was a strong family man who was in love with his wife and adored his children. This time, during the trance state, the physician heard Spiegel speak about his responsibility to his wife and children, and that if smoking caused him harm it would cause them harm. The man wept as he repeated this message during the trance. As Spiegel learned afterward, this experience put an immediate end to the doctor's cigarette habit.)

During the last quarter hour of the session the patient is again asked to go in and out of trance in order to fix the self-hypnosis procedure in his mind and to alter the eye-rolling, hand-in-the-air ritual so that it can be done in public without drawing attention. The eye roll is done with the eyelids closed and the floating hand is directed to the forehead so that it appears to be the familiar gesture of a person soothing a headache.

As he summarizes the strategy, Spiegel observes: "What you are learning here is, in essence, an art form. It is the art of learning how to control an urge. And in that connection, there is a basic principle: If you mean to control an urge, don't fight it." Fighting it only makes it worse. It is better to ignore it by devoting one's attention to another urge: the urge to respect your body. He tells an ancient Zen parable about a jackass tied by a long rope. "One end is around its mouth and the other end is tied to a pole. As long as it thinks like a jackass, it pulls and pulls. All it gets out of that is a sore mouth and a tighter knot. When it stops thinking like a jackass, it discovers it doesn't have to pull on the rope; and if it doesn't pull, the rope slackens; with the rope slack, it can walk around, lie down, go here, go there; and when the rope is slack long enough, even the knot gets loose."

Finally, to drive home his point about the innocence of one's body, he asks the patient what he would do if he had a pet dog and he opened a pet-food package bearing the warning, "The Surgeon General has determined that this food is dangerous to your dog's health." "Would you feed the dog that food? No? Then why not give your body the same consideration you would give to a dog?" He speaks of the care an adult takes in leading a child across a street. "If you look at your body as this trusting, innocent part of you, do you see how natural it can be to take a position of respect and protection toward your body?"

Inevitably, there are patients who are not at all impressed by Spiegel's approach. Some expect hypnosis to jolt them magically out of their cigarette habit and are disappointed to learn that the responsibility is on themselves. Some think his message about protecting the body is nothing more than a statement of the obvious. The urge to smoke is too powerful to be put down by platitudes, they feel, and so they keep on smoking. Or else, like the fashion editor from Memphis, they stop smoking even as they grumble about the "silly" and "tiresome" monologue.

Most people, however, take the message to heart. They give up smoking; some for a while, some permanently. But why? What happens in such a brief time that triggers a breakaway from a habit that may have endured for years or decades?

For some patients, hypnosis is the least part of it. Their motivation to stop smoking is genuine and strong, but they apparently need someone or something to show them a way out of the perceived trap of the habit. They are attracted by the notion of adopting a custodial attitude toward the body. The concept of the body as an innocent part of themselves, as deserving of respect and protection as a child or a favorite pet, may never have occurred to them. Simply hearing it for the first time can be enough to tip the scales and bring an end to their smoking. For others, hearing the concept while in the supremely attentive stance of the trance state makes it all the more intense and meaningful and memorable.

Once again, it must be said that the hypnotic trance is a very special state of mind. It magnifies the hypnotist's words (and the patient's own words during self-hypnosis). The message goes into the gut, so to speak, as the usual censors of the mind step aside, and it can take on the power of a strongly held belief. To make sure that the concept holds fast as an important new element of a patient's life-style, he is asked to do the self-hypnosis exercise periodically. By having something to do for himself instead of depending on a doctor to do it all for him, the individual becomes his own healer.

Very often, more is accomplished than the conquering of a destructive habit. There is a new and healthier attitude about caring for one's personal physical plant. A physician who stopped smoking after a session with Spiegel told him, "This may sound funny, but I used to treat my body like a rhododendron—you can get away with not watering it for a long time. Taking care of myself wasn't important so long as I thought I was okay. But now I look at it differently: There's two of us and we're friends."

Another doctor, a psychiatrist who attended the Columbia course, did not mean to quit smoking but did so anyway after being exposed to the discussion of the mind-body relationship. "I was profiled as a One-Two," he explains, "but because of what I learned I have changed a lot of my orientation from basically Apollonian to more Dionysian qualities. I seem to feel things more, as if I'm more in tune with what my body is telling me. There was a good deal of emphasis at the course on stop-smoking techniques that are used with self-hypnosis. Well, I was a smoker, a pipe smoker, and I didn't really want to stop, but then I would be walking along and suddenly find myself saying, 'For my body, smoking is a poison.' I'd stop and say, 'What?' Or else I'd be sitting with a patient in psychotherapy, puffing away at my pipe, and I would become aware of the sensation of smoke in a way that I had never thought of before.

"I was relating to my body in a very feeling way instead of my usual thinking way. I would also get images of Freud and the oral cancer that he got from smoking so many cigars. That would just come to me. And these sensations and images happened with such frequency that I decided, well, I won't smoke today, and I didn't, and I haven't smoked since then. That really taught me something about myself. I stopped smoking and I didn't even need to go into a trance or use an exercise to do it."

After hearing this account, David Spiegel called it "a great example of weaving in left- and right-hemisphere language. Something about the stop-smoking message made sense to your Apollonian side. At the same time you could sense your body saying that something's going on here that I'm not happy with. Your Dionysian responses teamed up with your Apollonian reasoning. That's quite a combination!"

13

MASTERING SYMPTOMS

It is much more important to know what sort
of patient has a disease than what sort of disease a patient has.

—SIR WILLIAM OSLER

There once was a bright, well-educated woman named
Sheila, the wife of a successful psychiatrist and the
mother of two children, who lived in a wealthy suburb of
New York. By all appearances, hers was the good life. In
reality, she was a virtual prisoner in her own home. Although free to drive away from the house any time she
wished, she would become panic-stricken at the mere
thought of being in an automobile.

Sheila was terrified by vehicles. If circumstances com-
pelled her to go on an auto trip she would drug herself
with Valium first and always insist that her husband
travel only on back roads. Even then the journey would
be such a nightmare that frequent stops had to be made
so that she could find temporary relief from nausea, diar-
rhea, severe muscle spasms, and overall high anxiety.

Her phobia was just one of hundreds of phobias that
afflict millions of people. To be terrorized by cats or tunnels or high places or (as in the case of Peter Sellers) the
color purple may be, in the words of novelist Julie Baum-

gold, "as irrational and as infantile as the 'monsters' in the closets of childhood, but think of that clutch in the coeliac plexus when a car skids, and imagine it as a habit, a way of life, a private horror movie that never stops."

Sheila had something in common with the veteran truck driver described in the *Washington Post* who inexplicably developed such a fear of driving that, as the final indignity, he was forced one day to cower in the trunk while his wife drove their car across the Chesapeake Bay Bridge. A businessman with a similar malaise was so enslaved by his fear of traveling that he did not dare leave his house even to attend his father's funeral.

After several years of expensive psychoanalysis to unearth the roots of her problem, Sheila realized that all she really cared about was getting rid of the problem. On the recommendation of her analyst as well as her husband, she took her phobia to Dr. Spiegel. Finding that she was a psychologically intact person of average hypnotic ability (a Two-Three), he showed her how to use her trance talent to float above her anxieties. He also taught her a self-hypnosis exercise to reinforce a novel concept about the automobile functioning as an extension of her body and thus being subject to her mind and muscles. The feeling of control that she might acquire by this method would be related to the experience of champion racing drivers who tell of becoming so fused with their vehicles that they can feel the road through the tires as if through the soles of their feet.

Although Spiegel encourages patients to let him know how things work out, he did not hear from Sheila again after that one forty-five-minute visit until nineteen months later. She sent him a long letter in which she described herself as "the new Sheila." Saying that she had thought many times of writing him, she reported that the results "were successful beyond anything I could have imagined. Although I stopped hypnosis myself after a rather short period of time, the phobia has disappeared. I take long car trips now with no discomfort, either emotional or physical."

Spiegel decided to invite her to the next session of the Columbia course so that she could describe how she had used her trance ability to eliminate the phobia. One of the first things she said when she appeared before the doctors was that she had driven herself to Manhattan, "something I could not possibly have done two years ago. If I had come here then I would have gotten up very early in the morning, checked the weather report five hundred times, and even if it was sunny I would be sure that there was ice on the highway somewhere. I would leave the house in terror and force myself to come by cab. Now I drive everywhere—in the rain, in the snow, day or night."

The phobia had begun, she related, when her husband was still in medical school. "This led to great tension with my husband even though he was very decent about all the disruptions in our life and the fact that we rarely could go out anywhere." In addition to analysis, she had tried to deal with her phobia with acupuncture. "I believed in it, but it was a disaster. When I tried hypnosis, I didn't believe in it but it worked."

It worked because Sheila, as she employed her trance talent to internalize her new viewpoint about cars, had learned to float instead of fight. A phobia is a devilish trap. It is like the simple Chinese device made of entwined straw that fits over a finger: the more one tries to pull free, the more tightly it binds. Sheila became adept at putting down anxiety attacks by shifting into a relaxed trance state. She could float going to the car; she could float driving in the car. She was able to function with the kind of calm assurance that is far safer on a busy highway than the panic-stricken mood of a driver who is fighting himself as well as the traffic.

When she asked Spiegel during her appearance at Columbia whether she could use her hypnotic ability to deal with another but less disrupting phobia—her dread of high winds and rainstorms ("It's a part of the reason we moved from the shore to the woods")—he took the opportunity to guide her into trance and teach her the screen technique. By going into hypnosis when a storm begins, she could separate herself from her fears by projecting them on her private movie screen. "You don't have to deny the anxiety, but you can examine it and negotiate with it more effectively if it's out there on the screen and not here where it gets you all uptight."

One of the most frequent comments made by clinicians who learn hypnosis from Spiegel is that his therapeutic ideas, especially restructuring, are every bit as valuable to them as his information and insights about hypnosis. The common thread of his strategies is the news that something can be done, starting now; that it is the patient who will be the prime mover in effecting a change or a cure; that the patient has within himself the resources to deal with his affliction; and that there is a new way of looking at the thing that has held the patient in its grip for months or years.

For phobics, insomniacs, stutterers, teeth grinders, hair pullers, fat people, shy people, migraine sufferers, victims of performance anxiety, and all manner of other people who are afflicted by one thing or another, the very idea that something can be done—that order can be brought to the chaos of their lives, that they can take charge of themselves—will itself give propulsion to the treatment strategy.

For the smokers mentioned in the preceding chapter,

the treatment called for a fresh perspective about respecting and protecting their innocent bodies. For those individuals who are afraid of flying, to take one of the better-known phobias, the new outlook they are urged to accept is directly related to the notion of the-automobile-as-an-extension-of-your-body that car phobics like Sheila are encouraged to adopt.

Even though commercial flight is considered the safest way to travel, millions of Americans have never flown because of aviophobia. Their numbers are so great that some airlines sponsor group therapy programs. The typical course for flying phobics teaches relaxation techniques that amount to simple hypnosis without the label. Passengers are taken, step by step, through a familiarization process that helps them understand what holds the airplane up and to feel ever more comfortable near a plane and in a plane. Finally, they go aloft on a graduation flight.

The high success rates claimed by the better-known programs are the product of multiple treatments. Spiegel uses restructuring with hypnosis in a single session and apparently gets results that are as good or better. "Of all the clinical syndromes that we see for one-time treatment," he says, "the success rate for flying phobia is the best. It is better than for cigarette smoking, better than for pain, and far better than for obesity. Although we aren't sure why, our two- to seven-year follow-up studies indicate that the best achievers are intact people in their forties with an eye roll of two-three or above and a better-than-high-school educational level." With this one-time approach, two out of three of the patients who can fully use their trance ability—those with intact profiles—succeed in flying comfortably.

One of Spiegel's more memorable patients was a former Korean War paratrooper who had jumped twenty-two

times into enemy territory and won the Silver Star. "Ten
years later he came to me because he had been afraid of
flying ever since he came home from the war. He told me
that when his plane landed in San Francisco, he suddenly
panicked because he realized he didn't have a parachute
on. He had been used to jumping out of planes with
a parachute, not landing in planes without one. He
couldn't believe his panic. He said he looked at all his
medals to assure himself that he was not a coward. But
when he got on the connecting flight to New York he
became a white-knuckle flier, fighting his terror all the
way across the country. When he staggered off the plane
in New York, he said to himself, This is it! He knew he
would never set foot in another airplane. But eventually,
when he got to be the vice-president of a corporation, a
job that involved a lot of traveling, he realized that he
would have to fly or find some other line of work. He was
under acute stress. When I showed him how he could use
his trance capacity to put himself into a whole new relationship with the airplane, and to float above his fears, he
got over his terror. He's been flying ever since."

Spiegel's fear-of-flying strategy, developed over a number of years, was influenced by Marshall McLuhan's contention in his book *Understanding Media* that "for the
first time man has become aware of technology as an
extension of his physical body." The strategy's essential
ingredient, however, came to Spiegel much earlier under
most unusual circumstances. In the North African desert
in 1943, while being transported to a hospital in a jeep to
have the shrapnel removed from his leg, he saw an American P-38 pilot who had just been wounded in an air battle parachute to the ground and land nearby. The pilot
was picked up and taken to the hospital with Spiegel.
They became great friends. One day the pilot told of how
terrified he had been when he first learned to fly and how

his fear had vanished as soon as he stopped "fighting the plane" and started to see it as a machine that was a part of him because he had such control over it.

When Spiegel sees a fear-of-flying patient for single-session treatment, he tells him that behind the fear "you are unconsciously fighting the plane. This is absurd. The plane is a mechanical instrument that is neither for you nor against you. You can correct this misconception by feeling yourself floating with the plane. Float with the plane, feel the plane as an extension of your body; by floating with the plane, you are correcting this fear.

"All of man's instruments are, in effect, an extension of his body. For example, if you want to pound something into the ground you can use your fist. You can also use a hammer. In that sense, a hammer is an instrument that is an extension of your body, your arm, your hand. If you want to point, you can use your finger and arm. Another way you can do it is to use a wooden pointer. In that sense, the wooden pointer is an instrument that is an extension of your body. If you want to go from here to there, one way to go is to walk. Another way is to use a bicycle. In that sense, the bicycle is an instrument that is an extension of your body, your legs. Still another way to go is to use an automobile. In that sense, the automobile is an instrument, an extension of the legs. Still another way to go is to fly. The airplane is an instrument that in effect is an extension of the body. You can make this connection by feeling yourself floating with the plane. *Float with the plane!* In the course of floating with the plane, you are simultaneously ignoring and dissolving the fight with the plane, and, as a consequence, the fear."

The patient is taught the same twenty-second self-hypnosis exercise that the smoking patient learns but the message that is reimprinted is the concept of floating with the plane. He is told to practice the exercise periodically during the day in preparation for the flight, and then to do it en route to the airport (at a traffic light, for example), and in the terminal, and while going to the plane, and in the plane.

During the flight, Spiegel continues, the patient can remain in a formal trance throughout or he can reserve the trance state for the landing. He can also use the stepped-up imagination that is possible with self-hypnosis to envision the pilot as his personal agent so that "your hand through the pilot's hand on the instruments is in effect controlling the plane."

At the conclusion of the session, Spiegel asks the patient to meditate on the difference between a possibility and a probability. "Of course there is a possibility that the plane will crash, but it is highly improbable. The sign of a phobia is that you deal with a possibility as if it were a probability." It is possible, he says, for an air conditioner to fall on the patient's head when he leaves the building, but in going ahead anyway he has chosen between a possibility and a probability and has given himself the freedom to walk on the sidewalk. "The same principle applies in your decision about flying. To ask for an absolute, positive guarantee means that you are in a trap. It is impossible to get that, but what you can do is extend your usual mastery technique in making choices and apply it to your decisions about flying, as you do with everything else."

For those people who have been the prisoners of a phobia, achieving mastery can amount to a born-again experience. Consider, for example, Sandra Marcowitz. She had lived in terror of dogs for three decades. After Spiegel showed her how to counter the terror with her trance capacity, her life changed for the better in so many ways that she set down an autobiographical account of her transformation and sent it to him.

Dog phobia was a family thing, Sandra wrote. It was shared by her mother, brother, aunts, and cousins. "I existed, frozen, immobilized by deep feelings of fear, shame, and embarrassment, because of my phobia and phobic behavior. Every waking hour of my life was spent planning my strategy of survival. As a child, if unaccompanied by an adult in the street, I searched out doorways and other escape routes from unleashed dogs. I waited on each landing until it was safe to run into my apartment. Childhood memories of afternoons without friends. Memories of the embarrassment of being different. Mocked by the kind of cruelty only children are capable of. Party dresses, but no parties. Suppose there was a dog at the party? I couldn't bear the consequences."

So she stuck close to home, sheltered by her books and music. She forced herself to go to school but she was "the personification of the silent student who knows the answer but never raises her hand in class. I was a shadow person, an observer but never a participant. Consequently my marks never reflected my knowledge. The information was frozen in my mind because I had to concentrate my energies on plotting the walk between home and school." Going home, "I knew which streets had the least number of unleashed dogs. I knew the streets with the most accessible doorways for ducking into for momentary safety."

This was the pattern of Sandra's life. She would be told that there was nothing to be afraid of, that the dog was more frightened of her than she of it, but "These were worthless palliatives because I knew intellectually that the dog would not harm me but I could not deal with it emotionally." Her fear of becoming an emotional cripple was almost equal to her fear of dogs. On one occasion, she forced herself to go to Mexico alone to see if she could function independently in a new place. She ended up staying in her hotel room most of the time, leaving only to take taxi trips to museums.

Although she went on in the next decade to carve out a semblance of a normal life, including marriage and a job, her unabating terror of dogs obliged her to concentrate on creating a "safe world" for herself. Finally, she found in her brother "the emissary of my emancipation from fear" because he sat down with her to discuss the reasons for the "family phobia." Apparently, it had all begun generations before in Eastern Europe. "I was told that dogs were used punitively to ghettoize the Jews. My grandmother left Rumania when she married my grandfather and brought the fear with her." Years later, "on seeing a dog in the street, my mother would run with my carriage."

Sandra's talks with her brother inspired her to seek professional help. Spiegel was recommended. "I proved to be hypnotizable [a Two-Three] and during the first session Dr. Spiegel explained my phobia to me as a normal progression considering my family background. He explained that I had never learned about domesticated animals. He taught me autohypnosis and a set of suggestions and steps I could take in my own time to overcome my phobia. He taught me the technique to gain *executive control* over my phobia and, consequently, my life. Through autohypnosis I was able to open up a part of my mind previously closed to receptivity about dogs.

"The plan was for me to arrange to work with a dog and follow a number of steps for which I would prepare myself daily through autohypnosis. The poodle next door, Dolly, became my cotherapist. For two days prior to my first planned encounter with Dolly I used autohypnosis ten times a day. I began each trance state with the following suggestion: My natural feeling of love and protection will enable me to overcome my fear of dogs. I asked Dolly's owner to hold her on a tight leash with the dog facing away from me. I was afraid of approaching her face-to-face so I started by stroking her back. It took me more than ten minutes to cross the room and touch her.

"Each day thereafter, I programmed myself through autohypnosis. The next steps were to stroke her whole back and head. It took me one week to accomplish this goal.

"Around that time my father visited my home. I was eager to demonstrate my ability to pet the back of a leashed dog. Just as I was about to do so, he uttered encouragingly the dreaded words of my youth, 'You have nothing to be afraid of.' I froze. I was unable to resume the first simple step. Once again, I knew intellectually he was right but his statement devastated me. The next day I saw Dr. Spiegel and he reinforced the hypnotic suggestion."

Because of the difficulty of arranging "dog time" with her neighbors, Sandra was given a puppy by her ex-husband. She promptly named it "Spiegel." The dog was confined in a large chicken-wire playpen in her apartment until she could go through progressive steps: "to have Spiegel lick my hand; to put my arms around Spiegel; to allow Spiegel to come to me—unleashed—for that final, all-encompassing hug of acceptance."

She said that she was "cured of a thirty-year phobia within one month." She felt as if she had been released from prison. "I no longer had the phobia but I still retained the habits of a phobic. For example, I had to learn to walk in the street without seeking escape routes. I learned 'dog etiquette'—how and when to approach dogs—because I wanted to touch and play with all of them! For the first time in my life, I walked the streets, parks, beaches, country roads or anywhere without fear of dogs."

Sandra's story ended with a detailed description of changes in her life because of her mastery of the symptom. The ripple effect was powerful. She no longer was obsessive about order and cleanliness in her home. Gaining control and mobility in her personal life reduced the need for regimentation at home. She was no longer preoccupied with books, films, plays, and art about concentration-camp victims and survivors. Her eating habits changed dramatically. Before the cure, eating had been "a joyless chore because I had a knotted, nervous stomach." She was reversing "thirty years of tension and tautness" in her body. No longer immobilized, she decided to complete her college education and study for a Master's degree in social work. She was free at last not only of her lifelong fear but of the humiliation of having the fear.

For many other disabling symptoms as well as phobias, control is the big issue. The individual feels that he is under assault and has no weapons; he cannot control his personal environment. Using hypnosis as a framework and facilitator for an appropriate treatment strategy, Spiegel offers not magic but self-mastery. The first trance experience gives proof that the patient can assume greater executive control over his body than he had imagined.

For any number of patients who see themselves as pitiful creatures of habit, hypnosis can open the way to an escape route, but it has to be hooked to a treatment approach that is suitable to the individual's particular abilities and personality. A clinician who knows the meaning of the eye roll and who can do a hypnotizability assessment is in a position to tailor the therapy to fit the patient and to take account of the differing responses of those who are high, low, or mid-range on the hypnotiz-ability scale. The Lows, for example, are prone to fight the symptom while the Highs tend to deny the problem. The alert therapist will notice and make use of the Apollo-nian's manner of thinking before feeling and the Diony-sian's manner of feeling before thinking.

David Spiegel had a unique opportunity to compare the Apollonian and Dionysian styles when two young women in Massachusetts, unknown to each other, came to see him a few days apart with the identical problem: hair pulling. Each of the patients had developed the habit of yanking bits of hair out of her scalp during anxious moments. So much so that bald spots were showing. They looked a mess and felt worse.

"Predictably enough," says David, "the Dionysian's way of dealing with the habit was total denial. She had started wearing a wig. That's a bad sign. It's supposed to keep the hands from yanking at the head but it just covers up the damage and the damage gets worse as the patient continues the habit instead of dealing with it. She responded immediately to the three-point strategy: that for her body, not for her, hair pulling was damaging; that she needed her body to live; that she owed her body respect and protection. She stopped the hair pulling com-pletely within three days. Then she wanted me to treat her as a psychotherapy patient. It turned out that she had a number of problems that the Highs often get. She was in a very destructive relationship with a schizophrenic law-yer who had threatened her with a knife one time and a shotgun another time. But she felt she didn't deserve any-one better. She got into intensive therapy and finally ended that relationship.

"The other young woman, who was referred by a group therapist, was a One. You couldn't find a more Apollo-nian person. She was preoccupied with the reasons for the hair pulling. She said it was a way of getting at her knotted nerves. She would do it when she was trying to work out math problems. She got me into such a debate about the existence of free will that I couldn't even do a complete Profile at the first session.

"The next time she came in, I said I didn't want to hear another word until we did the Profile. Then we went to work on a strategy for mastering the habit. When she turned up again three weeks later, she proved that she really had the mind of an Apollonian when she handed me a chart with a bar graph for every day since she had begun using hypnosis. The bars showed that her hair pulling was down some days by 60 percent, compared to pre-treatment hair pulling, and up 10 percent other days, but overall she was tapering off very well. She proudly informed me that she didn't do it exactly the way I said it. Modifying the exercise made it hers, not mine, but of course the advantage of this approach is that it leaves room for the patient to tinker with it, and the Apollonians usually will. This patient took about four times as long defeating the habit as the Dionysian but each was able to employ the restructuring concept in a different way on her own terms."

Meanwhile, back in New York, Herbert Spiegel was helping a patient with an equally nasty habit, except that the habit had persisted a lot longer. The patient was a handsome young attorney, cultivated and fashionably dressed, who chewed on his hands whenever he was tense. By all appearances, he was tense very often. He had been gnawing away at his hands ever since childhood, and now they were so unsightly that he kept them in his pockets or behind his back or concealed by gloves when he went out in public.

Telling himself to stop biting his hands did no good, he said, because while reading or watching television, for example, they would go into his mouth without his realizing it. (Says Spiegel: "That's the equivalent of a spontaneous, unstructured trance state.") After three years with a psychiatrist and after fruitless efforts with medication and assorted therapies, he was directed to Dr. Spiegel. "But," said the lawyer, "when I heard that this was going to be handled in one session, and then I was going to carry on myself with self-hypnosis, I almost didn't go. I was skeptical. It was too glib, too simple. I couldn't believe it when it worked. It worked so well that I went to one of Spiegel's medical lectures to show the doctors how I put myself in a trance for a few seconds every so often to remind myself that hand-biting is an insult to my body and that I need my body to live and I owe it this respect."

While such a habit for many another patient could have been conquered completely and permanently, this man was less successful. "After half a year there was a little slippage. I wasn't used to having fingernails. I would pick at them when they itched, and then I started biting again. I had already stopped the hypnosis, telling myself that the dialectic was the important thing, but in retrospect I realize that hypnosis was important for making me concentrate and being more receptive to what I was doing."

Spiegel saw the lawyer again to help him revive his control, but "the need for a reinforcement session," as he said when he reported the matter at the Columbia course, "suggests that this is one case that probably requires introspective analytic therapy.

"Usually the generating cause of a problem becomes unimportant as time goes by and the symptom remains as a kind of residual that can be directly turned around by the strategy we use. When that happens, then fine. But sometimes the very issues that generated the symptom in the first place—probably having a lot to do with family relationships in the case of this patient—are *still* critical, and they show themselves by undermining the new mastery. That's the message. It means that it is almost mandatory that the patient have a better understanding of what is the energy behind this. Once he understands it, I don't think there's any doubt that he will be able to control it. He has already demonstrated that he *can* control it. But we can see some kind of obsessional preoccupation about something that is going to take some analyst a lot of detective work. He tells me that since our second session a month ago he has not been biting his hands, except for one occasion, but, look, I think we're dealing right now more with his Apollonianism—since he is an admixture of Apollonian and Dionysian traits—and unless he gets some cognitive exploration and an understanding that satisfies him, I don't think he's going to maintain his mastery of this again."

In his more exasperated moments, Spiegel will half-jokingly declare that analysis is useful only for teaching analysts, but, as the foregoing case suggests, he concedes that it still has its place. What troubles him is the eagerness of all too many psychiatrists to go exploring for causes before trying to dispose of the patient's problem by the quickest route possible. Many of his colleagues in the profession, like others in all branches of medicine, behave as if they have never heard of hypnosis. Even those who learn hypnosis have to be restrained from going too far in treating a patient who simply wants to be cured of his most pressing and oppressing affliction.

During one address to a gathering of psychiatrists, Spiegel presented a thirty-five-year-old man who had telephoned him a few days earlier to see what could be done about his severe stuttering problem. The patient had agreed to be treated in front of the doctors instead of in Spiegel's office. There would be no fee. The patient explained to the audience that his affliction made his work as a businessman much more difficult. "As for my social life, it's a disaster." He went on to say that "the stuttering is at its worst when I talk to my mom. Talking to her on the phone is the worst of all." He had started stuttering when he was six years old. "At any time that I began to stutter, my mother would slap me in the face."

Spiegel's comment on this was the lighthearted observation, "If it isn't one thing, it's a mother." Maybe, he said, the patient is right in linking his mother to this problem, and maybe not, but it was not something he intended to pursue. "I'd rather pay attention to what is doable." When several psychiatrists in the audience pursued the matter anyway—one of them asking about the role of the man's father—Spiegel turned them off, saying, "I don't think it means a damn thing one way or another. The patient may have a hypothesis about this but he can't rewrite history. When he masters this thing he can take another look at his hypothesis if he wants to. What's important now is to get him off the idea that he's a vocal invalid. What we're saying is: Why don't you join the rest of us who can speak without stuttering? And here's how to do it."

Once therapy begins, Spiegel encourages a stuttering patient to see himself as a person, not as a stutterer. "As a person, you have many attributes and one of them is that you have somehow not been in touch with your natural rhythm. This has affected your speech. Now, if you want, we can put you in touch with your beat."

In the case of the businessman, he followed Spiegel's directions so well that in a matter of minutes he was speaking without stuttering, apparently for the first time since childhood. His own look of astonishment was matched by the expressions on the faces of the more skeptical observers in the audience. He was not cured;

there was a lot more practice that he would have to do on his own. But, as in learning to ride a bicycle, doing it once, however awkwardly, is to be on the way to doing it easily and forever.

Spiegel says that a stutterer may sound as if he is speaking slowly and haltingly but actually he is rushing headlong into speech and stumbling as he tries to make too many sounds at once. Spiegel's therapeutic approach is built on the work of Dr. John Paul Brady, head of the Department of Psychiatry at the University of Pennsylvania Medical School. Although generally he looks askance at gadgets and gimmicks, preferring to have his patients rely on their built-in capacities, Spiegel shows stutterers how to use a metronome to help them adjust their speech to a beat. Instead of bunching up their words in sudden bursts of speech, they deliver them in time with the metronome. The instrument can be dispensed with once the beat is internalized.

Until he gains control over his speech, the patient is expected to take twenty seconds or so every hour or two to slip into trance in order to—in Spiegel's words—"reinforce the concept of floating and at the same time remind yourself to speak and think and talk and feel in terms of the beat, the beat, the beat, always the beat. When you come out of this self-induced exercise, give yourself the posthypnotic signal that you will continue to think and talk in terms of the beat, the beat, the beat, always the beat."

Spiegel says he is amazed that this technique is not better known. "I have had patients who spent years and years with speech pathologists and going to special schools, making practically no progress, and in one session with this they've corrected their speech permanently. All stutterers are not the same, of course, but this is the best method I've ever come across. When I first read an article Brady wrote about it I got mad at myself. I used to ask my stuttering patients to imagine they were singing, because I was impressed with Jane Froman. She was a severe stutterer but she never stuttered while singing. In fact, I had never heard of anyone stuttering while singing. But it never occurred to me that there's a difference between the melody and the beat. It's the beat that counts. If you stick with the beat, you're okay. If you analyze most fluent speakers, they all have a beat. Brady puts his finger on it."

Stuttering is one of a number of conditions that are suitable for short-term therapy with hypnosis because they can be turned around quickly: the stutterer can start speaking clearly; the hair puller can stop pulling his hair; the smoker can become an instant nonsmoker. But some conditions do not have a sharp on-off, either-or character, and the most prominent and frustrating of them all is that all-American malady, obesity.

Because the overweight patient has to eat in order to live, the treatment goal is not to stop eating; the goal is rational eating instead of irrational eating. The usual approach by therapists is some kind of behavior modification. However, smart eating, as opposed to dumb eating, calls for such a fine tuning of an individual's everyday urges and habits that it is hardly surprising that there are no impressive long-term results for even the most prominent weight-loss programs.

"This country is full of people going on diets and crash diets," Spiegel says, "but these are short bursts of activity without any deep, long-range commitment. The experts who have studied diet programs have concluded that, overall, the success rate five years later is about 5 percent. So you have a multi-billion-dollar diet industry that is 95 percent ineffective in the long run. I had a patient who told me that on her latest diet she stuck to the rules so well that she would go to dinner at the finest restaurant in town and scarcely touch the food. But then she would rush home to gorge herself on Oreo cookies. In our approach we don't tell a patient what to eat or when to eat. That falls into line as soon as there is an acceptance of responsibility for one's body and a commitment to treat it well."

Spiegel's method for treating eating disorders, which takes far less clinical time than other techniques, may well be more effective than most, but he is quick to point out that his success rates for smokers, phobics, and others are much better. Patients who are within 10 percent of their ideal weight do very well, but those who are grossly overweight may have to be seen for more than one session, and even then a goodly percentage will start backsliding at some point in the future.

Dr. Harold Wain, the pain specialist at Walter Reed Medical Center, is now slim and trim, but he once was a fat man. He continued to be a fat man even after taking Spiegel's course and using hypnotic strategies with many of his patients, including those with weight problems. "But you're the one with the weight problem," his wife would tell him. "How can you charge the prices you do with your forty-inch waist and your stomach hanging out over your belt?" His customary reply: "But I love to eat!" Wain finally became so embarrassed by his corpulence that he used Spiegel's strategy with self-hypnosis to take off fifty pounds in five months and reduce his waist size from 40 to 34.

"When I ran into Dr. Spiegel at a conference in Montreal," he says, "he didn't know who the hell I was. He said it was like talking to a different person. I still love eating and I do eat well, but I've become a connoisseur instead of a common sewer. And that's what we stress at Walter Reed when we teach self-hypnosis for weight reduction. The theme is self-mastery and the necessity for each patient, while doing the trance exercise, to think of himself or herself no longer as a human garbage can but as a connoisseur, and to relish each bite of food and think of the increased enjoyment gained by cutting down on quantity."

For overweight patients, as with smokers, Spiegel's emphasis is on the opportunity to put an old problem in a new perspective—that of the person's relationship to his body—and to use the trance state to lock the new viewpoint in his mind. In periodic self-hypnosis exercises of relaxation and reflection, the patient reminds himself that overeating is a poison for his body, that he needs his body to live, and that he owes his body respect and protection. He is encouraged to reacquaint himself with his body so that when he meets it at his ideal weight, it will be like a reunion with an old friend. "Having prepared yourself for the meeting, you will be in a position to hold on to that friendship indefinitely."

What Spiegel asks of the fat man or the fat woman is a truly radical change in thinking about food and the human body, not just a change in eating behavior. "You are committing yourself to the idea of respecting your body and caring for it as you would care for your favorite pet if the veterinarian told you that it was important to control his diet. It's a lifelong engagement."

All therapy, of course, must fight an uphill battle against the emotional forces that in many instances produce the bodily symptoms. A limb paralysis or a facial tic may well be a somatic metaphor. And the more hypnotizable a person is, the more likely that his outside will express the turmoil going on inside.

One of David Spiegel's patients was a young woman who experienced great difficulty moving one of her legs after a close friend in college, in the course of a fatal illness, had a leg amputated. This same patient had so many other symptoms, including severe itching that stemmed from her anger at a man in her life, that David concluded that "her high dissociative capacity became a vehicle for her to express all kinds of conflicts and to confuse the hell out of physicians and for them to confuse the hell out of her." Once aware of her high trance capacity and the special features of her Dionysian personality, she was able to master her symptoms and reduce her vulnerability in human relationships.

Another patient, who happened to be lower in trance capacity but who proved to be highly motivated to cure himself, was a forty-three-year-old bricklayer whose left index finger had been fractured when an old ladder collapsed on his hand. Just prior to the injury, his employer had removed two newer ladders that he had been using on the job. Even those sturdier ladders were a poor substitute for the safer scaffolding that, in his opinion, should have been provided by the company.

The bricklayer was an angry man as he was given initial treatment for the fracture. Soon afterward, the index finger and then the three adjoining fingers curled tightly into the palm. There they became fixed in such a rigid position that the hand appeared to be permanently deformed. Although there was no physical reason for his inability to move his fingers, he could not do so. His all but useless hand prevented him from returning to work.

The bricklayer showed signs of anxiety and depression. He had been a regularly employed craftsman for twenty years, but now, with the loss of his job, his self-esteem hit bottom. Even though he received workman's compensation, his standard of living dropped sharply. He became involved in a series of lawsuits against his employer and the manufacturer of the ladder. Because of the litigation he was seen by several psychologists and psychiatrists, one of whom accused him of malingering. And because of the compensation issues involved, he was secretly filmed—as he eventually learned—to see if he was faking his inability to extend his fingers. When amputation of his index finger was recommended by one doctor, he refused.

As described in an article in *The Journal of Hand Surgery* by David Spiegel and a Stanford surgeon, Dr. Robert A. Chase, "The patient was caught in a situation in which a variety of health professionals had, in essence, attacked his integrity. To recover physically became the equivalent of admitting the premise of these evaluators that he was deliberately feigning illness. On the other hand, continuing the disability might conceivably lead to amputation of his index finger and to a continued demoralized living situation with reduced income and self-respect."

David Spiegel and Dr. Chase did not see this patient until long after the accident—three and a half years. Treating the contracture as a combined physical and psychological symptom, and sensing the importance of the man's wounded pride, they used the Hypnotic Induction Profile to determine that he had a moderate potential for experiencing hypnosis. (His depression may have accounted for the "soft" pattern of his one-two score but any difficulty he might have in reaching his trance potential could be offset by his apparent strong motivation.)

The bricklayer learned that he could help himself with self-hypnosis—using the trance state numerous times during the day to develop trembling movements in the hand that would increase gradually. He went about it with such enthusiasm that there was no doubt about his desire to recover from his affliction. Soon he was squeezing a rubber ball as an additional exercise. Eventually a splint that worked like a spring was attached to the index finger to help it extend as fully as the other fingers. Because the fingers had been curled rigidly for so long, therapy was prolonged, yet in less than a year there was virtually a full range of motion in all fingers and the patient was working again at his craft. His depression had long since lifted.

The key to success in this case, the two doctors believe, was the identification and use of the patient's capacity and desire for change, "transcending the adversary relationships which had been established between the patient and a variety of health professionals. Hypnosis was not used to challenge the 'reality' of his contractures, but rather as a rehabilitative device to enable the patient to master his disability."

A number of the health professionals who examined the bricklayer over the years were aware that psychological forces were at work, yet most of them seem not to have understood that, in all likelihood, there was in the patient's possession a remedial power that could be switched on at any time: his ability to shift into an altered state of consciousness and concentrate his mental and physical energies on one thing of importance. In many instances, doctors give no thought at all to psychological forces and remain blind to even the most obvious somatic metaphors.

Take the case of a young woman named Alice who had no history of skin disorders, yet who one day suddenly and inexplicably experienced such a terrible itching sensation that she rushed home to rip her clothes off. Soon she was covered from head to toe with a vast and unsightly rash. Nothing she did and nothing her doctor tried could make it go away. For two and a half years she wandered from dermatologist to dermatologist, and from hospital to hospital, in search of a cure. Her case became so famous among skin specialists that when she called on one dermatologist, his first words were, "Oh, you're the one!"

"I was forever being tested," she relates. "I couldn't believe I had that much blood in me. I've lost count of the names and the number of drugs I was told to take. They told me I had everything from Bell's palsy to arthritis. The day I went into the last hospital my face was beet red. I'd been having this redness and terrible heat in my system. My skin was now like dust. When I took my clothes off it was just like another body falling off me. The whole thing was flaking. I was screaming and crying when they put me in the dermatology ward. I was so thin that nobody I knew would recognize me. My hair and my eyebrows were falling out. They took so many biopsies that I thought they were making a new body. I never saw so many doctors. They had me on sleeping pills and antihistamines and other things that I felt were only making matters worse. I was hallucinating a lot. For about two months I lost track of time. When I came to, I was furious. Lying there, I heard my voice but I didn't recognize my body. When I looked in the mirror, seeing this person with no hair and the strangest skin, I thought, this isn't me, this is someone else."

Alice's husband suggested hypnosis as something to try, but the specialists said it would do no good. Finally, when all the experts had reached a dead end, the resident in charge of the case telephoned Spiegel to describe the problem and report that "we are beginning to suspect that there might be some psychogenic connection." Spiegel, who could not take on the case at that time, recommended Dr. Stanley Fisher, then a research psychologist at Columbia University's School of Public Health. Having studied hypnosis under Spiegel, he regularly directs workshops for physicians at the Columbia course.

"When I first saw her," Fisher recalls, "Alice was in bed, apparently sleeping. Her eyes were open and all white—the ultimate eye roll. I was excited because here, it seemed, was a highly hypnotizable, probably very emotional Dionysian, and it is well-known, though apparently not to all dermatologists, that many skin disorders are caused by emotional troubles. When she woke up, I did an evaluation. Even though they had her loaded with drugs, she scored as a straight Four.

"Whatever the reasons for her rash, the first thing was to get rid of the agonizing itching. When she told me that a soothing shower was the only way she had found to get relief, I taught her how to use her trance capacity to visualize being in a shower, having the water pouring down all over her body, and so on. Her whole body responded to that. When she was in trance you could see her body reacting to the cool, soothing water of the imaginary shower."

That first experience with self-hypnosis and her newfound ability to take charge of her body marked the beginning of the end of the rash and the itching and scratching. She was able to sleep soundly for the first time in years. Within days she was out of the hospital and within weeks her skin was back to normal.

But what about the causes? Her case was so extreme that Fisher felt it might help if they tried using her trance capacity to get some information. Alice was agreeable. He guided her into trance and suggested that she go backward in her mind to the time when the rash first appeared.

One piece of information that surfaced during age regression was that Alice had allowed her employer and co-workers to take advantage of her compliant nature and overload her with work. She had become tense and exhausted. But then some further data emerged that Fisher describes as "truth stranger than fiction."

Alice began to speak in a soft, anguished voice about her love for Nipper. She was "my adorable little black dog, fifteen years old." But the dog had become sick. "She was driving my husband crazy. He said I should get the dog put away and that it was my fault that something was wrong with her. I began to feel it was my fault. I tried to do everything. I kept bathing her and walking her—everything so she wouldn't scratch." But the scratching got worse and the dog became so sick that it had to be destroyed. Alice was the one who had to make the arrangements. "I felt awful. The vet even asked me if I wanted to hold the dog while he put her to sleep."

Because of this exploration, there was every reason to believe that the trauma of her dog's sickness and death, and the guilt feelings she felt after assisting in the dog's execution, were mainly responsible for the rash that burst forth at that very time. The dog's scratching became her scratching. As a Dionysian, she could be expected to express her feelings through somatic symptoms. With self-hypnosis, she learned how to control such responses.

When Spiegel met Alice one day, he said to her, "What would you think if I said to you that I absolutely disagree with you; that you weren't responsible for your dog's death?" Her reply: "That's been told to me, but I still feel it."

"The lesson here," says Spiegel now, "is that for all the plasticity and malleability of highly hypnotizable people, there is still a hard core that seems intractable in many ways. This is a reminder that hypnosis may be able to do something as dramatic as curing a symptom like skin rash, but it does not necessarily change everything. We can't always change everything or explain everything. Yet every time I feel frustrated, as a psychiatrist, about how little we know, I think of the dermatologists and a lot of other doctors and then I feel better."

14

PAIN

The strain in pain lies mainly in the brain.
—DAVID SPIEGEL

Edgar Allan Poe's headaches were so severe that he would rush outdoors to bury his head in the snow. Lewis Carroll is said to have written parts of *Alice's Adventures in Wonderland* while hallucinating during a migraine attack. John F. Kennedy, according to his brother Robert, was in pain from his many ailments, injuries, and operations "at least one-half of the days that he spent on this earth." Sigmund Freud suffered constant pain during the last seventeen years of his life as cancer ate its way through his jaw and palate. Shunning all drugs except for an occasional aspirin in his final days, Freud told a friend: "I prefer to think in torment than not be able to think clearly."

Pain is personal. It is an unsharable experience. No one else can feel the pain we feel. Not even the smartest doctor with the most sophisticated equipment can confirm that the pain is as terrible or as tolerable as we say. Pain is something that everyone knows about, but no one fully understands. The experts are still trying to explain the "phantom limb" phenomenon: the aching that an amputee may feel in a hand or a foot that no longer exists.

Pain, real or imagined, can be a convenience: "Not tonight; I have a headache." It can be rewarding: "My son calls me every day." A patient receiving disability payments may be less motivated than others to get rid of the hurt in a hurry.

More often than they know, people create their pain. On the eve of Appomattox, General Ulysses S. Grant, tense and anxious as he awaited word of General Robert E. Lee's response to his peace proposals, experienced such a blinding headache that he had to take to his bed. He was still in agony when a messenger arrived with the good news that Lee was willing to discuss the terms of surrender. To Grant's astonishment, as he noted in his diary, the pain in his head disappeared.

As the complaint heard most often by physicians, pain is commonly seen as an enemy; yet, over the course of human history, sages have spoken of pain as a teacher and friend who gives us the truth even if it hurts. Pain tells us to drop the hot frying pan. A toothache delivers the message that it is time to visit the dentist. "Pain is part of the body's magic," Norman Cousins has written. "It is the way the body transmits a sign to the brain that something is wrong."

In recent years there has been so much interest in pain that it can be described as a veritable growth industry. Pain has become one of the most popular of the medical specialties. New drugs, surgical techniques, and electronic devices have appeared as fresh weapons in the endless war against suffering. Pain clinics and pain control centers have sprung up at medical institutions all over the country. There has been great excitement about the discovery that our brains contain natural analgesics called "endorphins" that are, milligram for milligram, much more powerful than morphine. A number of researchers, having concluded that we produce these natural narcotics to combat pain under traumatic conditions, believe that endorphin production explains acupuncture, the placebo effect, and perhaps even hypnotic pain relief. However, one of the pioneer investigators in this field, Dr. Avram Goldstein of the Addiction Research Foundation in Palo Alto, has cautioned physicians and scientists not to go overboard on the endorphin theory of pain. David Spiegel has been working closely with Goldstein and his associates on a clinical study that shows that hypnosis can alleviate pain without altering endorphin production.

To Herbert Spiegel, the endorphin research suggests that there is more than one way in which people negotiate pain: "I've seen nothing to cause us to change what we have said so far about hypnosis and pain. If there is anything to the endorphin hypothesis, it involves a different order of pain reduction and is unrelated to psychological effects."

When speaking of pain, which he has described as "an urgent call for action" from the body to the mind, Spiegel emphasizes the all-important difference between pain and the way we perceive pain. The pain signals that reach the mind through the nervous system are one thing; the way the mind processes the signals is something else. "It is useful to think of pain perception," Spiegel says, "as a complex interaction between the physical stimulus that causes the pain and the psychological reactive component to it which we call the hurt." The physical stimulus can be so severe, as in the case of a crushing blow to some part of the body, that the perceptual apparatus is overwhelmed and the psychological factor is minimal. But if the pain is less intense, as in most clinical situations and in most instances of chronic pain, "the reactive component is important and provides great flexibility in the perception of pain."

The medicine men of primitive cultures appear to have understood the psychology of pain better than many of today's highly trained physicians. In his *Book of the Eskimos*, Peter Freuchen describes the Eskimo healer, or *angakok*, as an expert in the art of trance who inspired belief and had a suggestive influence over his patients. "In this way," Freuchen writes, "pain frequently disappeared, as the patient was hypnotized into feeling well. Once, when I was assisting in the amputation of some broken fingers, the injured man felt no pain because an old sage sat by him speaking pain-dulling magic formulas during the operation."

Similarly, James Esdaile's patients felt no pain (or, more precisely, ignored the pain they felt) because of the "mesmeric trance" that he employed in hundreds of operations in India in the mid-1800s. "But since Mesmer had been declared an impostor," writes Arthur Koestler in *The Art of Creation*, "medical journals refused to print Esdaile's papers." In 1842, Koestler adds, a surgeon named Ward "amputated a leg painlessly under hypnotic trance and made a report to the Royal Medical and Chirurgical Society. The Society refused to believe him. One of its most eminent members argued that the patient had merely pretended not to feel the pain, and the note of the paper having been read was struck from the minutes of the Society."

Pretending not to feel the pain of an amputation is, of course, a wondrous achievement by itself, as the eminent member seems not to have realized. In fact, make-believe is one of the factors at work when hypnosis is used to counter pain. The pain remains—and may even be revealed by facial expressions during the trance—but the patient either refuses to acknowledge it or overcomes its impact by directing his mind to more agreeable things. He *chooses*, in other words, not to let the pain hurt.

Unfortunately, most of us do not know that we have a choice. And yet everyday life gives us innumerable examples of the mind's ability to take pain or leave it. There is the child who stops bawling about a bruised knee when his attention is diverted by candy or a game; the youth who shrugs off an injury in order to impress a girl friend with his manliness; the prizefighter who cannot be bothered to feel pain as he concentrates on beating his opponent.

Spiegel tells of a young mother who heard a scream as she backed her station wagon out of her driveway and realized that she had struck her five-year-old boy. She found him pinned under a wheel when she ran to the back of the car. "Although weighing less than 120 pounds, she lifted the corner of the station wagon in the air, enabling a neighbor to pull the child from under the wheel. She rushed him to the hospital. Only after she was told by the doctor that the boy's injuries were not serious did she notice a pain in her back. X rays of her spine revealed that she had fractured three vertebrae in the process of lifting the station wagon. There can be little doubt that the accident elicited a trance state in this mother, who focused so intently on the business of rescuing her child that she totally dissociated her own self-inflicted injury until the mission was accomplished."

Such spontaneous, unconscious pain control calls on the same inner resources that are mobilized by hypnosis. It is entirely within the capabilities of most people to "filter the hurt out of the pain," Spiegel says. Milton Erickson observed: "One can always forget pain. One of the things that I don't understand about patients is why they continue to keep their tension and pain."

David Spiegel tells this story about himself: "I was

going to England, and it was a terrible flight. I arrived at Heathrow airport with a splitting headache. I put my first shilling into an aspirin machine at the airport and the damned machine didn't work. Then I got on the bus for London and we were bouncing all over the place. The headache was getting worse and worse. Halfway to the city I said to myself, 'You idiot! You teach people how to use hypnosis for pain control and you forget about using it for yourself. For God's sake, do it!' So I sat there and put myself in a trance on the bus. In five minutes the headache was gone. I couldn't have been more surprised."

Mid-range hypnotic subjects like David and his father do not have the ability of highly hypnotizable persons to set aside pain sensations completely even in the most extreme situations, but they can make the most of the trance equipment they have. "When I go to the dentist," says Herbert Spiegel, "I focus on a feeling of numbness, like giving myself a shot of mental Novocain. I can still feel the touch as he is drilling the teeth. I am aware of the grinding. It is not an absence of pain; it's just that I can negotiate the pain without making a big fuss about it. I was in a labor room once with a woman who was using hypnosis for the delivery. She obviously was having contractions—you could see the strain on her face—but her attitude was, as she said, 'I know I have the pain, but the hell with it.' "

Although Spiegel received the usual medical-school instruction in the nature of pain, it was not until his combat days in North Africa that he fully realized the importance of the patient's attitude about the pain he feels. Even before receiving his own disabling wound, which he found strangely easy to take, he had observed in the field hospitals that many of the wounded soldiers were almost blasé about their pain, as if saying that it was a small price to pay, after their close encounters with death, for the pleasure of being alive.

"Sometimes they didn't even know they had been hit until the battle was over," he recalls. "One of our best officers, an engineer who was assigned to the infantry, was a very gung ho, highly motivated guy who was hit in the right shoulder blade by a shell fragment. I saw it and picked out the fragment. The bone was fractured. When he saw my aide filling out a tag to send him to the rear, he asked, 'What are you doing, doc?' I told him he was wounded. He denied it. I told him to try moving his arm. When he couldn't do it and realized that he had been hit, this big, strong officer broke down and cried."

Later on in the war, another army physician, Dr. Henry K. Beecher, was serving as an anesthesiologist with the hospital unit at the Anzio beachhead when he noticed that the combat casualties required far less morphine than had been expected. This observation eventually led to Beecher's classic study of pain patients. He compared the pain experiences of 150 of the Anzio wounded with those of 150 surgical patients at Massachusetts General Hospital. The many complaints of the hospital patients and their demands for medication stood in sharp contrast to the reports of minimal pain by the soldiers and their modest requests for medication. Beecher concluded that the civilians regarded pain as an altogether unrewarding interference with their everyday lives, whereas pain to the soldiers was almost welcome as a sign that they were alive and on their way to making an honorable exit from the war. And since remaining alert would help insure their survival, the soldiers had little desire to have their mental processes slowed down by drugs.

"Any small boy in a fist fight," wrote Beecher in the *JAMA*, "feels no pain at the time of injury. This comes later, when his bloody nose begins to drip or his mother arrives to console him. The severely wounded soldier, not in shock but clear mentally, has surprisingly little need for a narcotic. In the early hours after wounding, only a minority request it, whereas the civilian recovering from surgery with a much smaller wound receives two or three times as much narcotic as the soldier with his more extensive wound."

Pain is what we make of it. Or, as Beecher concluded, "The intensity of the suffering is largely determined by what pain means to the patient." Some people refuse to let pain of any kind put them down; others succumb to the first pang. Some cultures encourage people to weep and wail and cry for help when pain strikes; other cultures make it clear to everyone that pain is nothing to make a great fuss about. True believers of certain religions show their faith by their stoic acceptance of pain. Distance runners, weight lifters, competitive swimmers, and other athletes of the more strenuous sports welcome pain as a confirmation of their dedication and as a measure of their progress. In his book about conquering the four-minute mile, Australian runner Herb Elliot told of his coach's instructions to "thrust against pain" and to "love and embrace suffering."

The importance of attitude and motivation in pain perception was understood by the late Dr. Ralph V. August, a Muskegon, Michigan, obstetrician who was well known in medicine for his use of hypnosis in 85 percent of the thousands of vaginal deliveries he performed as well as in two thirds of the cesarean-section deliveries. He said of hypnosis that it "allows maximum comfort for the mother with a minimum of sedation for the infant." Dr. August also noted that recovery is faster. When the *JAMA* asked him about instances when hypnosis did not work well in childbirth, he recalled that it was ineffective in the case of "a mother whose divorce was pending and in a mother who was bearing an unwanted child."

One of the features of Spiegel's Columbia course for many years has been a remarkable medical film of Dr. August at work, *Hypnosis as the Sole Anesthesia for Caesarean Section*. Endorsed by the American College of Surgeons, it has been seen by thousands of doctors all over the world. The patient in the film is a young woman, relaxed and cheerful in her hypnotic trance as she responds to Dr. August's suggestion, "Your mind seems to be floating on a cloud as you look down on your body." He encourages her to sing her favorite songs as he operates, saying that the more she sings, the less the discomfort. He also asks her, from time to time, to describe the colors of an imaginary crystal ball. She does so enthusiastically. There is no hint of childbirth as an ordeal. Blood flows as Dr. August makes his incision but his patient sings merrily. She sings more loudly as he brings out the baby with head clamps. She beams when the child is shown to her. When she hears crying, she exclaims, "That's my baby!" She is still smiling and singing and describing crystal-ball colors as the doctor closes the incision.

Some years ago, Australia's foremost expert on medical hypnosis, Dr. Ainslie Meares, decided to find out for himself what it was like undergoing surgery with only the protection of a hypnotic trance. As he reported in the *Medical Journal of Australia*, Meares persuaded a dental surgeon to let him use self-hypnosis during a complicated tooth extraction.

The surgeon had to do an incision of the gums, remove the bone over the third molar with a bone chisel, thus exposing the roots of the tooth, and then pull out the tooth with forceps. Meares told the surgeon that he would raise his arm if he wanted the dental work to stop—"to allow me to regain my relaxation"—but he said afterward that the thought of raising his arm never occurred to him.

"I was aware all the time as to what was going on but the awareness was rather vague. When I realized that the bone was being chiselled and that I was not experiencing any pain, for the moment I felt myself becoming angry, as I thought that I must have been given an injection without my knowing it. I then realized that I would not be deceived in this way, and my momentary anger passed off. During the actual extraction I was aware of what was happening and experienced some sensation in that area. This sensation might possibly be described as pain without the hurt of it. There was practically no bleeding. There was not a spot of blood on my handkerchief when I returned home. After the extraction I was surprised at the completeness of the anesthesia, and the thought came to me that I might experience some after-effect. However, I had no after-pain at all. When I arrived home I remember trying to assess my mood, and I decided that I was neither elated nor depressed, but quite normal in my mood and comfortable in myself; and in fact I took my family to dinner at a restaurant and spent the evening at the theater with no discomfort in my mouth whatsoever."

One of the most vivid descriptions of a trance experience during major surgery was provided to Dr. Spiegel and Dr. Ernest E. Rockey by a fifty-year-old cancer victim. His ability to use hypnosis creatively saved his life. The man had come to Rockey with a cancerous lobe on his right lung. It could only be removed by a three-hour operation. That appeared to be an impossibility, however, because his extreme emphysema ruled out general anesthesia.

"Most doctors would have said, leave the man alone

and let him die in dignity," Rockey says, "but I knew he could go into a deep trance and I decided to go ahead with hypnosis." Because Rockey was still new to hypnosis at the time and uncertain about the staying power of a three-hour trance, he asked Spiegel to join him in the operating room and help him devise an effective trance strategy.

Just before surgery began, Spiegel guided the man into the trance state. He suggested to him that he was in a bathtub filled with ice. The ice would cool and numb his chest. Rockey, scalpel in hand, simply added, "Feel yourself floating in ice water surrounded by ice cubes." Then he began to cut. Because of the parallel awareness of hypnosis, the patient remained attentive to Rockey's occasional reminders about feeling an icy numbness while contentedly dwelling for three hours in some frosty, painless place of his imagination.

The operation went beautifully. Afterward, Spiegel asked the patient what he could remember of the procedure. "First I felt as though my windpipe were frozen," he said. "Then I felt him marking my chest with a pencil and I wondered why." In fact, the "pencil" was Rockey's scalpel. "Anyway, from then on I don't remember a damned thing. The next thing I remember is coming into a recovery room."

Spiegel rehypnotized the patient in order to get more details. This time he said: "I can remember a sort of crunching sound—I expect my ribs were being cracked. I could hear it. Then I remember floating in the Arctic, watching an iceberg with seals and penguins and things like that. I was trying to make a joke of the whole thing. That was the idea, to create a chilly situation." He said he was glad things had worked out so well because "I'm a coward when it comes to pain."

Long and complicated operations with hypnosis as the

sole means of stifling pain are obviously not for everyone. Only 5 to 10 percent of surgical patients would be able to forgo chemoanesthesia altogether in such circumstances. More would be able to succeed with hypnosis alone in less strenuous procedures. Most often, hypnosis is employed in association with chemoanesthesia, not as a replacement for it. The more a patient can float through surgery and tune out the pain signals, the less medication he needs.

When he sees people with pain problems, Spiegel first satisfies himself that no further medical explanation of the cause of the pain is required. The typical patient has been under a doctor's care, but still the pain persists. There is a strong desire to avoid dependency on painkilling drugs and to resume normal life.

After determining the patient's trance capacity, Spiegel spends a few minutes discussing pain perception. He points out that an individual can influence pain by controlling both muscle tension and the amount of attention that is paid to the pain. Very often, people produce even more pain than exists in the first place by tensing the muscles around the painful area. To demonstrate this, Spiegel asks the patient to "make a tight fist, stretching out your arm straight. Now, make a fist three times harder than that, and concentrate on the pain you feel as a result of this muscle tension. Now, let the fist open, and notice how the pain from the muscle tension dissipates."

The patient is then asked to produce pain by pinching the web of skin between his thumb and forefinger. "All right, now stop, and let the pain go away. Now try it again, the same way. Only this time, look at that painting over there on the wall and tell me what you think the artist was trying to say." More often than not, the patient will report that he felt less pain while trying to figure out the painting. He realizes now that shifting his attention away from the pain can actually reduce its impact.

Spiegel varies his treatment strategies for pain patients according to their trance capacities. Since an Apollonian is less able than others to handle the hurt with his imagination, the strategy is to put his mind to work on a distracting stimulus. "Each time you begin to feel the discomfort," Spiegel might say, "focus instead on the exquisite sensations you can feel in the fingers of your left hand. Rub your fingers, one against the other, and describe to yourself the texture, the temperature, the sensations, that you feel. Each time you are tempted to concentrate on the sense of discomfort elsewhere in your body, rub your fingers together gently, and discipline yourself to pay attention to the sensations in the fingers in your left hand. This becomes an exercise through which you filter your perception of the pain and concentrate instead on what you choose to."

Spiegel recalls one elderly Apollonian who succeeded in mastering his pain very satisfactorily except for a brief period after lunch each day. "This really intrigued me. It turned out that he had been in the habit of taking a nap after lunch. Since hypnosis is an alert state of concentration it follows that it's more difficult to concentrate when you're tired. He would become fatigued every day after lunch and feel the pain. But after finishing his nap he had no trouble using hypnosis to take care of the pain, right through suppertime. Then he took a bit of medication before going to sleep. So, with this combination, he was able to go on with his life quite comfortably. One of the lessons from this is that you don't tell a patient that he's not going to have any more pain if he uses hypnosis. That would be absurd. A doctor who says, 'When I touch your body, the pain will go away,' may provide temporary relief but the patient will feel cheated as soon as the hurt comes back. What you do is teach people to control the pain to the extent of their abilities."

In a typical session with a Dionysian patient, Spiegel might say: "Imagine yourself sitting in a dentist's chair. Picture the lights in the room, the feeling of the chair, the smells and sounds of a dentist's office. Remember the time when he took out that large needle and injected Novocain into your gum. Try now to re-create that feeling of the pressure in your gum and the gradual numbness spreading throughout your jaw and your cheek. Feel your cheek getting more and more numb, that numbness spreading throughout cheek and mouth. And then when you are ready, let your hand float up and touch your cheek and feel how numb it is. As you feel that numbness, let the numbness spread from your cheek to your fingers so that your hand begins to feel numb. Then let your hand float over to touch the part of your body in which you feel some discomfort, and let that numbness spread. This numbness becomes a filter through which you experience pain, and you learn in this manner to filter the hurt out of the pain."

Although an Odyssean cannot be expected to imagine numbness with quite the facility of a Dionysian, he may well be able to employ the metaphor of temperature change during the trance state to ease his pain. Most people, Spiegel finds, associate coldness or warmth with pain relief. They can draw on their memory of a soothing experience—a cold shower, a warm breeze—to make the self-hypnosis exercise more effective.

"While your hand is in the air," Spiegel might say to the Odyssean patient during trance, "imagine yourself floating, and as you feel yourself floating, make it more vivid by imagining that you are floating in water. Make it ice water. As a matter of fact, make it so icy that you feel the cubes of ice floating in the water, and as it gets colder and colder, you can even feel an imaginary tingling numbness coming from the cold. This tingling numbness gives you a protective coating around the pain area, so you learn to filter the hurt out of the pain."

Like the Apollonian and Dionysian patients with their own self-hypnosis routines, the Odyssean patient is encouraged to practice this brief exercise, which takes about twenty seconds, every one or two hours. If the patient tops off each trance episode with a posthypnotic signal to retain the feeling of numbness, he should be able to experience pain relief around the clock, in and out of trance.

"Even though intellectually you know that the pain is there," Spiegel explains, "by making your commitment to the imposed numbness, you feel the numbness more than the pain." Just in case the patient should find himself becoming more aware of the pain between the self-hypnosis exercises, he is taught how to use a private signal to reinforce the commitment to the feeling of numbness. The signal might be the clenching of a fist or the stroking of the pain area or another part of the body.

All of these elements of hypnotic pain relief can be used by the patient in his own fashion—and on his own schedule, for whatever length of time—as he finds them effective. Since the idea is to make pain control an integral part of one's life-style, Spiegel is not at all disturbed if the patient modifies the suggested trance strategy. This is something an Apollonian is much more likely to do than a Dionysian. He recalls a patient who was very successful at controlling his head pains. "I had taught him how to relax by imagining himself floating in water. When he came to the Columbia course as a guest to talk about his experiences, he said, in front of the audience, 'I don't want to hurt your feelings, doctor, but floating in water doesn't work at all. So what I do is float in grape Jell-O.' "

A frequent and almost predictable by-product of hypnotic pain relief, and of other trance exercises, is the telescoping of time. There is nothing mysterious about this. In everyday life, waiting for a bus will seem like hours if one is standing alone in the rain on a street corner; but the wait will seem like nothing at all if one's mind is focused on an animated conversation with an old friend who happened to be passing by.

One of Spiegel's patients was a woman who had developed metastases of the lung and spine as well as a gastric ulcer eight years after undergoing a mastectomy for breast cancer. Because she had found the necessary gastroscopy—the examination of the interior of the stomach—to be incredibly painful, he taught her to use her trance talent to imagine a long ice tunnel in her body from her mouth to her stomach so that she would experience a numb and tingling sensation instead of the usual pain. She called him after the next gastroscopy to report that the ten-minute procedure, which on previous occasions had seemed to last much longer, was now accomplished in two or three seconds as far as she could tell.

"When the doctor took out the tube," she said, "it was so short a period that I thought something had gone wrong and they would have to do it over again." But then she realized that it was her own doing—the result of her turning on her powers of mind. "This is the greatest thing that has ever happened to me. It has made my hospital stay almost enjoyable. I know I have some kind of control in myself that I was never aware of."

15

FUTURE TRANCE

> Compared to what we ought to be, we are
> only half-awake. We are making use of only a
> small part of our physical and mental re-
> sources.
>
> —WILLIAM JAMES

Many months ago, when I set out with Dr. Spiegel on a
journey into the country of the mind, retracing the steps
of his explorations of the last four decades, my intention
was to discover for myself what hypnosis is and is not,
and to be able to say how we might use it to enrich our
lives. Now, at journey's end, I find that the true value of
hypnosis is not so much in the uses to which we put it as
in the understanding it gives us of the powers of mind
that we scarcely know we possess.

In case after case mentioned in these pages, the great
unexpected bones of hypnosis is the revelation of un-
tapped talents and abilities. People speak of stepping outside themselves, of seeing themselves in a new light, and
of experiencing greater control over themselves than they
had ever known. In many instances, the ritual of hypnosis used to deal with a problem quickly becomes unnecessary as the mind takes charge of the body in a most
natural and routine way, as if it had been waiting all
along for just the right signal.

I believe it is telling that when Spiegel teaches hypnosis to doctors, he spends little time on the so-called art of trance induction and a great deal of time driving home the message that the mind matters in medicine, and that hypnosis, as a way of tapping the latent resources of the mind, is the cheapest, safest, most available, and often the most effective of all the means of healing.

A number of years ago, he was invited to lecture at a medical school in Jamaica where aspiring doctors from many Caribbean nations receive their training. "Here I was in a place where a lot of very effective healing has been done for centuries by what we dismiss as native mumbo jumbo," he says. "I found myself in the odd position of telling them to take a good look at their own medical tradition and perhaps use some of it, but I didn't make much of an impression. They didn't want to know about primitive ways of getting the mind to heal the body. They wanted *modern* medicine: drugs, surgery, hospitals, machines, technology."

Conversely, the experienced practitioners who take Spiegel's course at Columbia's College of Physicians and Surgeons are anxious to learn how hypnosis can help them in their work; yet some find it hard to grasp the essence of any ceremony that turns on an individual's trance capacity—that it is not what the doctor does *to* the patient but what the patient does *for* himself.

One day at the course, Dr. Pete Wolfe described an example of old-style, rapid-fire healing with an unsophisticated patient. She was a woman with a head tremor who had been under treatment with a noted neurologist, but the drugs he had recommended had failed to stop her head from shaking. Wolfe told her to bare her shoulders. Reaching for a pair of shiny acupuncture needles, he declared, "This is the way to stop the tremor!" Then he stuck the needles into her shoulders with the flair of a matador. The tremor disappeared. "That will be ten dollars, please," he said. The tremor was still gone when she returned for checkups a week later and a month later.

One of the doctors who heard this story missed the point. "You must know exactly where to put the needles," he said. Wolfe almost exploded. "No, I don't!" he roared. "It doesn't matter where the needles go! It's the patient's belief in their power that matters in acupuncture. The needles could just as well be a couple of pieces of gum. If the patient thinks they'll work, then they'll work."

I began this book with the observation that hypnosis, far from being an outdated and unscientific means for healing, may well be the most modern of all the tools of modern medicine. At the frontier of the mind, hypnosis starts where technology stops, and it is the mind that will be central to the medicine of the future. I also suggested that hypnosis has been reinvented, not just revived, and that the developments of recent decades have served to strip this much-misunderstood subject of its old authoritarian trappings and offer it as a self-mastering experience suitable to a free and enlightened society.

The myths and misgivings about hypnosis die hard, but brain research, biofeedback research, and the insights and discoveries of clinicians and university investigators have provided fresh knowledge of the power of the mind to influence the body. The creation of methods to measure hypnotizability and to match different trance capacities to corresponding treatment strategies has made the medical use of hypnosis far less of an unpredictable, hit-or-miss procedure. The idea of the patient as healer and the doctor as helper that lies at the heart of clinical hypnosis today is altogether in tune with the ideals of holistic medicine as practiced by increasing numbers of clinicians. There is every reason to believe that hypnosis in its modern form is on its way to becoming a part of accepted practice in virtually every branch of medicine. Two centuries after Mesmer, it is an idea whose time has finally come.

Hypnosis, of course, has applications outside of medicine. Amid much controversy, it is being used in law enforcement to search the memories of crime victims and witnesses. In education, experimenters have devised programs in "suggestology" to see if such elements of the hypnotic experience as relaxation, suggestion, and heightened imagination can lead to faster learning and more effective teaching. Self-hypnosis has been the prime ingredient of the assortment of self-awareness and human-potential ceremonies and programs that have been appearing—and sometimes quickly disappearing—since the 1960s. Such methods often promise more than they can deliver because they usually overlook the wide differences in mental functioning that are evident to clinicians who measure trance capacity.

Intriguing as it is to speculate about a future when forms of hypnosis are in widespread use for mind enhancement outside medicine, I have concentrated in these pages on hypnosis as a vehicle for healing. I have tried not to claim too much for it. Hypnosis is not for everyone. Some people are made for it, some are not. It is no cure-all. It comes with no guarantees. It is just one of a number of things a medical professional can employ to help a patient—or a patient can use to help himself. Several of the case histories cited have illustrated that motivation is often more important than hypnotic ability. Because of the many variables of any patient-therapist relationship, a trance strategy can sometimes work with patients who are incapable of trance. In fact, the third of the three principles that Dr. Spiegel sees as basic to hypnosis (see chapter 6) amounts to a disclaimer of exclusive properties and deserves repeating: "Nothing can be achieved in therapy with hypnosis that cannot also be achieved without hypnosis—except that in some instances hypnosis appreciably facilitates the time factor."

All this being said, it is also true that hypnosis frequently can work with stunning effectiveness when all else fails. Further, it is true for some people that the activation of their trance capacity can be a life-changing and even a lifesaving experience. There is high adventure—"the highest adventure on earth," Norman Cousins once said—in the unleashing of powers of the mind that help people achieve greater control of their lives. The irony of hypnosis is that a process or phenomenon that has been perceived by many as a means for one person to control another is now coming to be understood in terms of self-control and personal freedom.

When a patient tells a doctor, "I've got a problem," he really means, "A problem has got me." If a pain, a phobia, a destructive habit, a psychologically based ailment, or any other affliction remains impervious to conventional remedies, the individual feels trapped and helpless. He no longer is in charge of his life. If hypnosis proves to be the agency for his discovery of latent abilities to regain control, he has every reason to view it as a liberating force. Most of the cases mentioned in this book are the stories of individuals who unknowingly brought their own remedies with them when they sought help. "Each patient carries his own doctor inside him," Albert Schweitzer once said. "They come to us not knowing that truth. We are at our best when we give the doctor who resides within each patient a chance to go to work."

Sandra, the woman who became "a shadow person" because of her terror of dogs, and Sheila, whose fear of cars had made her a virtual prisoner in her own home, were able to use their minds to free themselves from the bondage of their terrors. A former paratrooper outwitted his fear of flying. A businessman stopped stuttering. A victim of seemingly uncontrollable convulsions discovered that she could turn them off before they started. A two-star general found that he was able to order away his agony. Terminal cancer patients controlled their pain so well that they dramatically reduced their use of drugs. A fashion editor suddenly called a halt to the slavery of a habit that had led her to smoke half a million cigarettes in thirty years.

I see the issue of control as central to the hypnotic experience. As Spiegel says, the paradox of hypnosis is that you give up control to gain control. You allow yourself to be influenced in order to achieve an extraordinary influence over your own processes of mind and body. You open yourself to new possibilities; you set aside your normal screens of critical judgment. What occurs in this singular state of mind—this dissociation from normal brain functioning, this business of being here and there at the same time—has much in common with the creative process that allows an artist or scientist to let his imagination soar. "The temporary relinquishing of conscious controls," writes Arthur Koestler in *The Art of Creation*, "liberates the mind from certain constraints which are necessary to maintain the disciplined routines of thoughts but may become an impediment to the creative leap."

It is perfectly possible for people to do remarkable things outside the formal hypnotic state—endure pain, accomplish incredible physical feats, perform amazing tricks of memory, imagine the unimaginable—but there is something about hypnosis that makes it all the easier. In *The Brain Revolution*, Marilyn Ferguson calls hypnosis "man's priceless practical joke on himself. Suspending his almighty judgment to comply instead with the hypnotist's instructions, he can heal himself, stand immobile on one foot for an hour, recall the names of the children in his kindergarten class—all feats no one with common sense would attempt in his right mind."

The ancient worry, of course, has been that if a hypnotist can talk a person into doing things he normally could not or would not do, what is to prevent an unscrupulous hypnotist from directing him to do something indecent or criminal? Many works of fiction are centered on the fear of loss of control during hypnosis, yet the reality of the trance state is that the hypnotized person is at the peak of control. In this alert and focused state of mind, he is at once responsive to directions and watchful and protective of himself.

One of the folktales out of classical hypnosis tells of the time that Charcot, the great French neurologist, appeared in a medical-school amphitheater to demonstrate hypnotic compliance. He customarily left the hypnotizing of his subjects to the medical students who served as his assistants. On this occasion, the assistants presented him with a young woman who was deep in trance. He handed her a knife and ordered her to stab to death a professor who was standing nearby. She obediently attacked the professor. No harm was done because the knife was, of course, made of rubber. Charcot informed the audience that the subject was under such control that she could not help but comply with every instruction she heard. Charcot then told one of the assistants to take the girl away and dehypnotize her. The medical student could not resist the temptation to suggest to her, while she was still deeply hypnotized, that it was evening, that she was preparing for her nightly bath, and that it was time to take off her clothes. Instead of stripping, the young lady snapped out of the trance, slapped him across the face, and stalked out of the room.

I heard John Kihlstrom, a Professor of Psychology at the University of Wisconsin and a leading hypnosis researcher, tell this story several years ago at a hypnosis symposium. "The lesson here is important," he explained. "The young woman knew that the great professor Charcot would not allow a murder to be committed before a big audience in a university auditorium. Knowing that there would be no consequences to the thing she was told to do, she obediently went through the motions. Later, with the medical student, she knew there would be consequences to what she was told to do. She was able to maintain control and not go through with the act."

Numerous experiments by investigators of hypnotic phenomena indicate that the subject does indeed maintain control even though in hypnosis the urge to go along with the hypnotist's suggestions is strong. If the subject is informed, for example, that his hands are stuck together as if bonded with glue, they will probably remain stuck together until the hypnotist removes the suggestion. The subject tells himself that he can free his hands if he wants to but somehow he does not want to. "In the hypnotic state," wrote a reporter after being hypnotized for the first time, "I was totally aware of where I was and completely conscious of the fact that I was in a state of hypnosis. I never felt incapable of stopping all this nonsense, but the thought of doing so was about as appealing as getting out of a warm bath on a sub-zero morning." If an unethical hypnotist, however, should suggest that his subject do something contrary to his customary moral code, that person almost certainly will end the trance and express his indignation. But it is also true that the trance state can serve to unlock inhibitions, much the same as intoxication or getting into the mood of a party or being swept away by the emotions of the moment. It can provide a convenient cover for exhibitionist behavior that a normally prim and proper person might secretly or unconsciously wish to carry out. He or she can always claim afterward, "I didn't know what I was doing," even if it is not altogether true.

The rule of thumb for hypnosis—that the real control is with the person being hypnotized and not with the hypnotist—needs to be qualified or clarified, of course, in the case of the Fours and Fives who shift into trance all too easily and deeply. One of Dr. Spiegel's most important contributions to our understanding of human behavior is the identification of the characteristics of the highly hypnotizable personality. We have seen in several chapters how the extraordinarily open, trusting, uncritical, and compliant tendencies of the Highs that can lead them to new heights of the imagination can also expose them to the possibility of exploitation and manipulation.

People with high eye rolls need to be aware of their proneness to trance and their vulnerability to influence in everyday encounters with others, Spiegel says. "Instead of learning how to go into trance, they have to learn how to stay out of trance." Charles Snyder, the highly hypnotizable antiques expert who took part in the *Fact or Fiction* experiment described in chapter 6, was asked during an appearance at the Columbia course whether he ever used his superior hypnotic gift to do his own age regressions or to probe his mind for buried information. "I have no reason to," he replied. "I'd feel I was misusing it. I want a medically sound reason. Dr. Spiegel gave me a tool to use when I have nightmares, whether awake or asleep. It has spared me hundreds and hundreds of nights waking up and crying in terror. One time I was in a restaurant and I felt very nervous for some reason. I felt like the top of my head was coming off. Then suddenly I felt very calm and there I was, sitting with my arm in the air."

Although my own commonplace capacity for the trance state does not come close to Snyder's extraordinary talent, I share his feeling of respect for hypnosis. I am often asked by friends and acquaintances who know of my work on this book whether my new familiarity with the subject makes me a hypnotist. In other words, do I go about hypnotizing people? Do I put on demonstrations or try to help people with their personal problems?

My answer is that I know enough about hypnosis and the human mind to know how little I know, and that I have too high a regard for hypnosis to use it foolishly or frivolously. I make a distinction between, say, helping an accident victim switch off the agony and doing hypnosis just to do hypnosis. Adventuring in another person's mind without being qualified to deal with unexpected reactions is a good way for an amateur hypnotist and his subject to get into trouble.

David Spiegel recalls the time he demonstrated hypnotic age regression with a student volunteer at Stanford. The young man was returned to his days as a three-month-old baby. "When I tickled him I expected him to giggle, but he burst into tears instead. This is not the time for a hypnotist to get frightened, because the subject can get frightened too and the thing will snowball. I just changed his age to six months and everything was fine. Later on, I asked him if he had had any health problems as a baby. He said his mother had told him that he had had a very bad abscess in his left chest when he was two months old. He had been very sick and was in the hospital for a month. And there I was, tickling him right where his abscess had been."

There is an obvious difference, of course, between a

reluctance to fancy oneself as a hypnotist and the exercise of one's personal trance capacity. In my own case, without any important medical problem that might benefit by the leverage of hypnosis, I have found that simply being conscious of hypnosis as a natural phenomenon can be every bit as worthwhile as the actual employment of hypnosis as a mind-shifting ceremony. Knowing my eye roll, knowing where I stand on the scale of hypnotizability, knowing that I do indeed have the traits and tendencies common to the Odyssean personality amounts to a considerable education in self-awareness. It is exciting to consciously shift mental gears so that I can, for example, move from an Apollonian mode of thinking to a more freewheeling and even reckless Dionysian style—and to know that this mixture of "measure and madness," as one writer calls it, is at the root of any creative exercise.

I realize today, as never before, that many ordinary uses of the mind resemble the parallel awareness of formal experiences with hypnosis. I mean in particular being totally focused on one thing of importance while somehow monitoring both my own performance and the surroundings. Like many other people, I can ignore all other talk at a crowded cocktail party as I engage in a conversation of my own, but if my name is mentioned in a far corner of the room I will hear it clearly. Moreover, I can do some long-distance eavesdropping simply by tuning out the person who is speaking to me. As a writer, I find that I am capable of concentrating so completely on the words before me that I seal off all distractions. There is no ringing telephone or roaring vacuum cleaner—not until I come out of my cocoon, and then the sounds rush in like the tide. At the movies, if the picture is worthwhile, I give it such undivided attention that I become emotionally involved with the characters and events.

Awareness of these capacities of mind has practical benefits. At the onset of a headache, I no longer reach automatically for the aspirin bottle. I know there is a better, safer way. The headache loses its hold and slips away as soon as I stop fighting it and start floating. At the dentist's, for routine procedures, I need only fantasize in order to filter the hurt out of the pain. While the dentist does his job, I take myself to the seventh game of the World Series and become so engrossed in my appearance at bat in the last half of the ninth inning that the dental work is done before I have a chance to hit the heroic home run.

Because of such experiences, such newly discovered talents, I no longer find myself puzzled by the cures at Lourdes, the ability of firewalkers in the Far East to go barefoot across a bed of glowing coals, and other phenomena that express the deeper resources of the mind. I also have come to see the significance of something that happened to me years ago in Japan.

At the time, as a foreign correspondent in Tokyo, I attempted to accompany President Kennedy's Secretary of the Interior, Stewart Udall, during a long day's climb to the top of Fujiyama, the snow-capped sacred mountain. Unlike Udall and the rest of his party, however, I was a complete novice at climbing. Within the first half hour of the ascent I was totally exhausted and due to collapse at any moment. I realized to my dismay that I would be unable to cover the story to the end. So great was my fury at myself that I just kept on putting one foot in front of the other. I became an automaton, mindlessly stumbling along the steep cinder trail far behind all the rest. My sense of detachment was so great that hours later I was only vaguely aware of passing Udall and the others as they sat on the narrow path taking a break. Some time afterward, euphoric beyond description, I found myself alone in the snow at the top of Fuji. I had time enough to get out my cameras and take pictures of everyone else coming up from below.

This was, of course, a profound trance experience. I know it now; I did not know it then. But I did get an early glimpse of inner resources that I had not imagined existed. Doubtlessly, many other people have been transported in much the same way. It is said that we use only a fraction of our mental power and that we go through life half asleep. Millions of people may think of hypnosis as some kind of sleep state, but if hypnosis is anything, it is our supreme way of waking up.

Brain researchers and investigators of altered states of consciousness foresee a time when most people, beginning in childhood, will know how routinely to achieve levels of self-mastery that we now associate with yogis, Zen masters, and a few other exotic figures who seem to have a knack that the rest of us lack. Apparently, we all have more of a knack than we know. Hypnosis in its ceremonial sense—an induction by a hypnotist or by the ritual of self-hypnosis—is a means for opening a window to the mind. How we go through that entrance is as much a matter of will and purpose as talent and temperament. Each step we take, however, is a step closer to our true selves.

"I can't believe *that*," said Alice in *Through the Look-ing-Glass*.

"Can't you?" the Queen said in a pitying tone. "Try again: draw a long breath, and shut your eyes."